Secrets Of A Healer - Magic of Massage

SECRETS OF A HEALER

VOL. VI
MAGIC OF MASSAGE

Dr. Constance Santego

Maximillian Enterprises
Kelowna, BC

Secrets Of A Healer – Magic of Massage
Copyright © 2020 by Dr. Constance Santego.

Copy Editor and Interior Design: Constance Santego
Book Layout: ©2017 BookDesignTemplates.com
Cover Design: Jennifer Louie

Ordering Information:
Quantity sales. Special discounts are available on quantity purchases by corporations, associations, and others. For details, contact the "Special Sales Department" at the address above.

Trade paperback ISBN: 978-0-9783005-7-9
Ebook ISBN 978-0-9783005-8-6
Created and published In Canada. Printed and bound in the United States of America

First Edition
Published by Maximillian Enterprises
Kelowna, BC
Canada
www.constancesantego.ca

*D*edication To
My first Massage Instructor, Harry.
May your legacy live on.

Allow your fingers to be your eyes.

– Dr. Constance Santego

ALSO BY DR. CONSTANCE SANTEGO

FICTION
The Nine Spiritual Gifts Series:

Journey of a Soul – (Vol. 1 Michael)
Language of a Soul – (Vol. 2 Gabriel)
Prophecy of a Soul – (Vol. 3 Bath Kol)
Healing of a Soul – (Vol. 4 Raphael)

NON-FICTION
The Intuitive Life, The Gift of Prophecy, Third Edition

Fairy Tales, Dreams and Reality... Where Are You On Your Path?
Second Edition
Your Persona... The Mask You Wear
Angelic Lifestyle, A Vibrant Lifestyle
Angelic Lifestyle 42-Day Energy Cleanse
Archangel Michael's Soul Retrieval Guide

SECRETS OF A HEALER, SERIES:

Magic of Aromatherapy (Vol. I)
Magic of Reflexology (Vol. II)
Magic of The Gifts (Vol. III)
Magic of Muscle Testing (Vol. IV)
Magic of Iridology (Vol. V)
Magic of Massage (Vol. VI)
Magic of Hypnotherapy (Vol. VII)
Magic of Reiki (Vol. VIII)
Magic of Advanced Aromatherapy (Vol. IX)
Magic of Esthetics (Vol. X)

FOR CHILDREN

I am big tonight. I don't need the light!

Contents

Preface xiii

Note to Reader xvi

Learning Outcome xviii

PART ONE..1

What is Massage?...3

History of Massage 5

Spa Massage vs Massage Therapy.....................7

Types of Massage...9

Benefits of Massage 13

Contra-Indications 15

    Contra-indication Subgroups.........................16

    Fixed Contra-Indications 17

    Flexible Contra-indications 19

    Other Important Considerations....................21

    Refusal to Massage......................................22

    Client/Practitioner Boundaries....................23

What Comes Next?...25

    Basic Anatomy and Physiology - Specifically for Relaxation Massage 30

    Muscle Chart 37

    Origin to Insertion......................................40

    Contraction...41

    Fiber Direction..42

    Fascia 43

    Anatomical Position.....................................45

    Movements of the Body 46

    Body Mechanics/Ergonomics.......................47

Client Care...52

Draping/Toweling...54

Your Mood 55

Massage Oil...56

Grapeseed Oil - *Vitis vinifera* 56

Olive Oil - *Olea europaea*.................................57

Coconut Oil - *Cocos nucifera* 57

Jojoba Oil - *Simmondsia chinensis*..................58

Castor Oil - *Ricinus communis*..........................58

Massage Table or Chair...64

PART TWO 67

Setting up for the Massage 69

General Rules to Massage..71

Basic Movements..72

Resting Position...72

Effleurage (Broad stroke) 73

Stroking (Broad and Intermediate stroke).....74

Pétrissage (Intermediate and Specific stroke)...........74

Compression (Intermediate stroke)...............75

Friction (Intermediate stroke) 76

Vibration (Intermediate and Specific stroke).............77

Tapotement/Percussion (Specific stroke) 78

Athletic Massage..79

Baseball 81

Golf...85

Hockey...88

Racket Sport-Tennis 92

Skiing/Snowboarding...96

Soccer...99

Swimming 102

Abdomen/Stomach Massage 106

Back, Neck, and Shoulder Massage 107

Breast Massage 114

Chair Massage 123

2 Minute Massage 124

5 Minute Massage 125

10 Minute Massage 127

15 Minute Massage 129

Facial Massage 132

Spa Facial 132

Hand Massage 134

Hot Stone Massage 136

Equipment Needed 137

Hot Stone Session: 139

Lymph Drainage Massage 142

Pregnancy Massage 147

Scalp Massage 153

Swedish Massage Relaxation Routine 155

Table Shiatsu 161

TIPS and TRICKS to having a pain free body 174

Bibliography 179

Message From The Author 182

Preface

The Miracle of Massage

I was late on the first day of my new job. Of course, I wasn't, but I was accused of being forty-five minutes late. To my surprise, as I opened the door to the practitioner's room and walked in, lying on the massage table was a lady with her breasts revealed.

Flabbergasted, I just did as I was told to do, copying what my mentor was doing. The rest of the day continued as a blur. That evening my husband asked how my first day went. To his astonishment, he heard me tell him that I started to learn massage, even though I was hired to work as a holistic counselor.

I had a paradigm shift that day. My career and life were never the same again. Instead, it led me down a magical path of integrated medicine.

It has been twenty-three years since that first day, and I have thanked God many times for the opportunity I was given to be taught by some of the most brilliant teachers in alternative medicine.

With an open heart, I go forward on my life's journey with gratitude and joy!

Enjoy, Constance

Note to Reader

Massage is not to replace modern medicine. Massage is for many purposes. Relaxation and stress relief improves the function of your body's systems, such as circulation and lymph drainage.

Unless your discomfort is muscle-related, it cannot heal you.

Your Doctor still plays a vital role in your health care. If I break my leg, I will need a Doctor and all the nurses and staff that work in the Hospital.

My understanding of Integrated Medicine is that **we play** a significant role in caring for our health. What we put into our bodies, how hard we work our bodies, the stress level we allow into our everyday life, and the positive or negative energy we attract around us all play a role in our wellbeing.

Shift happens...Create magic!

Learning Outcome

After completing this book and studying the concepts and techniques, you can perform many massages that help reduce stress, relax sore and achy muscles, and improve many of the body's vital systems, such as circulation and lymphatic.

- Relax, Rejuvenate, and Bond
- Many Different Types of Massages
- Be Able to perform Basic Massage Techniques on yourself, friends, and loved ones.

PART ONE

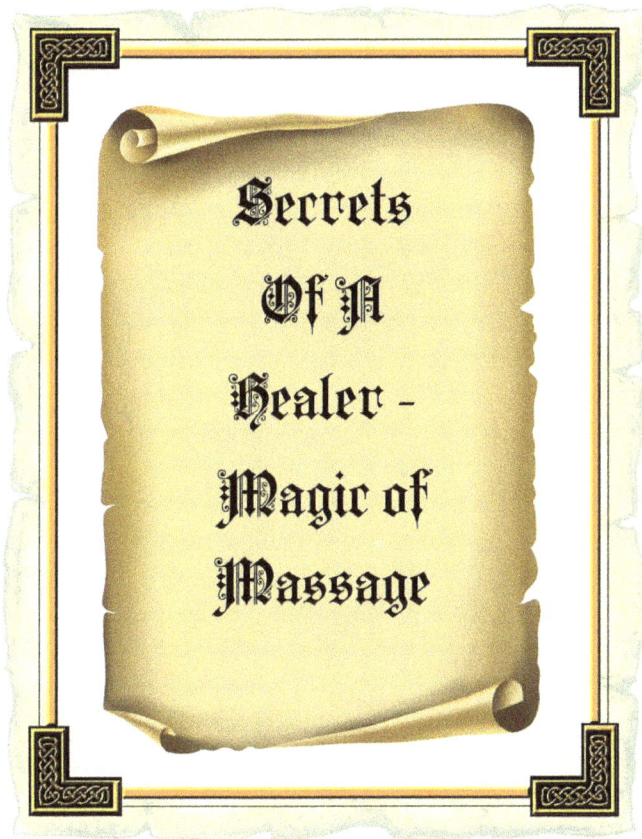

What is Massage?

Wikipedia Version:

Massage is the manipulation of soft tissues in the body.

Massage techniques are commonly applied with hands, fingers, elbows, knees, forearms, feet, or a device. The purpose of massage is generally for the treatment of body stress or pain.

My Version:

For over eighteen years, I practiced spa massage, aka relaxation massage, where the whole body is massaged. I usually started on the back, back of legs, front of legs, sometimes tummy, arms, head, and feet. I learned many, many different styles; European Lymph Drainage, Hot Stone, Chair, Aromatherapy, and Shiatsu, to name a few.

Deciding to learn more, in 2015, I graduated from the 2200-hour Massage Therapy program. The main difference is a client has a specific complaint, and the therapist addresses the areas of concern.

After I graduated, I combined my knowledge and practiced integrated massage. Using all the brilliant massage therapy techniques, I loved using specific techniques on the body to do the relaxation work.

In all the years I practiced massage, I found that if the problem was muscle related, I could fix the issues in one to three sessions. If it was caused due to a skeletal issue (a bone being out of place), I could only briefly relieve the pain, never fixing it. A Chiropractor usually is needed for that. If the issue was due to an accident, time and possible rehabilitation using a Physiotherapist were required. I could help, but I could not fix the problem.

Both Massage Therapy and Relaxation Massage are essential. In my experience, the person needs to destress—allowing the muscles to relax and heal.

Every client has different issues and should seek treatment from the appropriate professionals, not just because extended medical does or does not pay for it.

Receive the treatment you need; in many cases, it will be a relaxation massage to destress.

History of Massage

Ancient Civilizations

Once the great cultures and civilizations of the world started to develop, record-keeping became more critical. Early records report on massage and the different methods practiced at the time of writing. Examples include:

- **2760 BC** (*Approximately*) **Nei Chang** - a Chinese medical text was written that detailed massage procedures and their purposes.

- **800 BC** (*Approximately*) **Ayur-Veda** - an Indian book of wisdom and a collection of medical writings that describes massage.

- **460 - 360 BC Hippocrates** wrote extensively on massage for medical purposes.

- **131-201 AD Galen** wrote extensively on massage and described several ways it could be administered.

- **619-1279 AD Tang Dynasty** - masseurs were recognized as medical practitioners.

- The Japanese, Persian, Egyptians, and Greeks all recorded the use of massage.

Modern History

Although many of the ancient ways to heal were lost during the dark ages in Europe, they staged a renewal in the 16 and 1700s. Example include:

- 1518-1590 **Ambroise Pare**, a French surgeon, wrote about the effects of massage.

- 1700s **Hoffman and Guthsnuths**, two Germans, argued for massage and its benefits.

- 1776-1839 **Pehr Henrik Ling**, a Swedish fencing instructor, gained international recognition with the style of massage and exercises he developed.

- 1843-1913 **Just Lucas-Championniere**, a French physician, claimed massage was beneficial for soft tissues after a fracture.

- 1890s **English Surgeon, Sir William Bennet**, started using massage at St. George Hospital in London, England.

- 1984 Four women in England began a society of trained masseuses. They intended to raise the standards of massage and the status of women working in that field.

- 1900 The organization was incorporated.

Spa Massage vs Massage Therapy

Massage Therapists work on specific parts of the body. Relaxation Massage works on the whole body.

Massage Therapy is governed by many regulating bodies in Canada and the USA. As well, each province and state have its association and rules.

In Canada, as of 2013, a student must be granted the Diploma of Massage Therapy and complete and pass a minimum of 2200-hour program. In addition, to receive the designation of *Registered Massage Therapist,* a graduate must complete a government-approved provincial exam. Each province has its test requirements.

In the United States, each state requires anywhere from 500 to 1000-hour program needed to graduate.

Examples:

The BC College of Massage Therapy governs British Columbia Massage Therapy.

Alberta, Massage Therapy is governed by the Massage Therapist Association of Alberta and Natural Health Practitioners of Canada.

The American Massage Therapy Association governs California Massage Therapy.

SPECIAL NOTE: A Massage Therapist from a different province or state must pass that NEW area's board exam.

- o Estheticians, Holistic Practitioners, Natural Health Practitioners, or Day Spa Practitioners, you are <u>NOT</u> Massage Therapists.
- o You **cannot** legally **treat** a specific medical condition, whereas a Registered Massage Therapist can.
- o You **cannot** call yourself or advertise any title that refers to Massage Therapy, including Massage Therapist, Therapist of Massage, Massage Practitioner, or Practitioner of Massage. It is closely regulated, and doing so will create a civil claim, a fine, and the possibility of shutting your business down.

Types of Massage...

You may have received a massage and wished the practitioner applied more pressure, or maybe you wondered why it hurt so much.

The answer is quite simple. Every practitioner is different. They have different training, different desired outcome, and a different personal preference for the pressure to be used (softer to very firm). There is also a difference between a Spa Massage Practitioner – lighter pressure and a Massage Therapist – Deeper pressure.

A Massage Therapist is taught to treat a person's injuries or issues and cannot combine their practice with any other holistic treatment that is not accepted by their governing body, whereas a Spa Massage Practitioner is trained to do many different types of massages, mainly for pampering, relaxation, and preventative medicine. A Spa Massage Practitioner can combine the massage with many holistic treatments, such as Reiki or meditation.

THE MAIN TYPES OF MASSAGES:

- Aromatherapy Massage
  - o Adding therapeutic essential oils to the carrier used in the massage to help boost energy, natural healing, or uplift the spirits. The pressure applied is approximately 2 pounds.
- Aroma Scalp Massage
  - o Specific Techniques are taught to use on the head and scalp, and a personalized therapeutic blend of Essential oils is blended to stimulate your senses.
- Athletic Massage
  - o Using the techniques taught in the Swedish Massage course, a practitioner combines specific moves on specific muscle groups for each sport.
- Back, Neck, and Shoulder Massage
  - o Using the techniques taught in the Deep Tissue Massage course, a practitioner combines specific back, neck, and shoulder moves.
- Breast Massage
  - o Specific techniques and moves for lymphatic drainage. Excellent for cancer clients or preventative medicine.
- Chair Massage
  - o The client is clothed and usually sitting in a specially designed chair. This massage can be done using Swedish Massage techniques or Shiatsu pressure point techniques.
- Deep Tissue Massage
  - o Is used for the purpose of muscle, fascia, and connective tissue manipulation. It can

be excruciating for the client. The pressure applied is approximately 9-10 pounds.

- European Lymph Drainage Massage
  - o It is a precise massage taught to help drain the lymphatic system. Excellent for pre-post surgery, weight loss, relaxation, and after-competition sports.
- Hot Stone Massage
  - o The ultimate relaxation massage using heated basalt (lava) stones! But be careful. This massage has contra-indications (you cannot use it if you have some medical issues – if you can be in a hot tub submerged for twenty minutes, you should be able to have this massage).
- Pregnancy Massage
  - o An excellent massage to do on a pregnant woman during her whole pregnancy. Relief of muscle aches and pain, cramping, and swelling. The carrier oils help to prevent stretch marks.
- Swedish Massage
  - o We call this a muscle massage; it is used to stimulate the body to have more energy and to help relax those aching muscles. The pressure applied is approximately 4 pounds.
- Table Shiatsu
  - o Not considered a massage, the client is clothed and lying on a massage table for the entire session. It is excellent for improving flexibility and balancing the body's meridian system. The practitioner uses Chinese Medicine's knowledge of finger pressure (acupressure).

No matter what type of massage you have, the results should be beneficial for your body, mind, and soul relaxed muscles, extra energy, uplifted spirits, and, best of all, your body should feel balanced and rejuvenated.

Getting a massage benefits everyone, any time of the year; spring, summer, fall, or winter! However, if you are a massage practitioner, note that you will be busier in the fall and winter.

Benefits of Massage

The benefits outlined below may not all be gained by the massage taught to aromatherapists. The approach to massage takes in the emotional and mental as much as the physical.

The benefits of massage are:
- Mechanical
- Physiological
- Psychological

Mechanical effects of massage are the impact the massage has on the muscles. Skin, lymph, and circulatory system. Includes:

- Movement of lymph.
- Movement venous blood.
- Releasing and expulsion of lung secretions.
- Movement of edema.
- Movement of the digestive tract.

Physiological effects are often noted. Include:

- Increased blood and lymph flow.
- The increased flow of nutrients.
- Removal of waste.
- Encouragement of the healing process.
- Resolution of edema and hematoma.
- Increased extensibility of connective tissue.
- Pain relief.

- Increased joint movement.
- Facilitation of muscle activity.
- Stimulation of autonomic functions.
- Stimulation of visceral functions.
- Removal of lung secretions.
- Sexual arousal.
- Promotion of local and general relaxation.
- Reduction of stress responses.

Psychological effects are less obvious; however, the following have been identified as benefiting from massage:

- Physical relaxation.
- Relief of anxiety and tension.
- Stimulation of physical activity.
- Pain relief.
- The general feeling of well-being (wellness)
- Sexual arousal.
- General faith in the laying on of hands.

Contra-Indications

For the purposes of being able to define responsibility, the divide into two distinct groupings.

These are:

1. **Fixed Contra-Indications.** These contra-indications detail conditions of the body or mind that restrict the use of massage. You will not massage a client who has a fixed contra-indication. The only exception is when a physician has provided you with written approval and guidance. Then, only light massage with adjustments corresponding to the physician's direction can be used. An example would be a dying client. A physician may allow the massage to prevent bedsores, stimulate circulation, or enable the client to feel the touch during their last days.

2. **Flexible Contra-Indications.** The contraindications detail conditions of the body or mind that suggest that massage may not be appropriate or needs modification. The modification can be located, for example, not on a wound, below, or on varicose veins. It may be pressure, for example, very lightly on a pregnant woman's abdomen. It may be a change in routine or method or even cancellation of the massage entirely.

Contra-indication Subgroups

Both fixed and flexible contra-indications are divided into two subgroups. These are:

1. General conditions are usually not specific to or limited to a particular body part or location. While the condition may be in an exact location, it is more likely to be a disease or problem.
2. Local - conditions that are more specific to a body part or area.

Referral

If there is any doubt about the client's physical, mental, or emotional health, in all massage training, emphasis is placed on referring a client to a physician.

All assessment of the client is a means of discovering any condition that creates a contra-indication. If a condition's contra-indication massage is discovered, or a client states they have a specific condition that has a contra-indication, inquire if they have seen a Doctor or refer them to one before beginning a massage.

Fixed Contra-Indications

You will <u>NOT</u> massage a client who has a fixed contra-indication

General Conditions
Meaning the client is having this issue right now

1. Advanced respiratory failure
2. Anaphylaxis
3. Appendicitis
4. Asthma attack-severe
5. Atelectasis
6. Atherosclerosis severe
7. Cancer (non-terminal) Metastatic – *Need a Doctor's note first*
8. Diabetes with complications (gangrene, advanced heart or kidney disease, and unstable or high blood pressure)
9. Diabetic coma
10. Eclampsia
11. Epileptic seizure
12. Fever of 101.5 F or 38.3 1/2 C plus
13. Hemophilia - severe
14. Hemorrhage
15. Hypertension - severe
16. Insulin shock
17. Kidney failure
18. Liver failure
19. Myocardial infarction (MI)
20. Post-Cerebral-Vascular Accident
21. Post cerebrovascular (not stabilized)
22. Post myocardial infarction - unstable
23. Pneumonia - Acute
24. Pneumothorax
25. Respiratory failure

26. Shock – all types
27. Syncope
28. Systemic contagious/infectious condition

Local Conditions
Meaning the client is having this issue right now

1. An acute flare-up of inflammatory arthritis (e.g., rheumatoid arthritis, systemic, lupus erythematosus, ankylosing spondylitis, Reiter's Syndrome)
2. Acute neuritis
3. Aneurysms deemed life-threatening
4. Anti-inflammatory injection (24 to 48-hour post) target tissue
5. Arteritis -temporal
6. Burn-recent
7. Contagious condition -local
8. Ectopic pregnancy
9. Esophageal varicosities (varices)
10. Frostbite
11. Irritable skin condition - local
12. Malignancy
13. An open wound or sore
14. Phlebitis
15. Phlebothrombosis
16. Sepsis - a condition of
17. Temporal arteritis
18. Undiagnosed lump
19. Varicose
20. A wound or sore-open

Flexible Contra-indications

𝕸eaning you <u>may</u> under the Doctor's letter of approval or if they have had it but not now.

General
1. Any condition of spasticity or rigidity
2. Anti-inflammatory drugs, muscle relaxants, anticoagulants, analgesics, or other medications that alter sensation, muscle tone, standard reflex reactions, cardiovascular function, kidney or liver function, or personality
3. Asthma
4. Cancer
5. Chronic congestive heart failure
6. Chronic kidney disease
7. Coma
8. Diagnosed atherosclerosis
9. Drug withdrawal
10. Emphysema
11. Epilepsy
12. Hypertension
13. Immuno-suppressed
14. Inflammatory arthritis
15. Major or abdominal surgery
16. Moderately severe diabetes, juvenile-onset diabetes
17. Multiple sclerosis
18. Osteoporosis
19. Osteomalacia
20. Pregnancy and labor
21. Post CVA
22. Post MI
23. Head Injury

Local

1. Acute disc herniation
2. Aneurysm
3. Acute inflammatory conditions
4. Anti-inflammatory injection site
5. Chronic thrombosis
6. Buerger's Disease
7. Chronic arthritic conditions
8. Chronic abdominal/digestive disease
9. Chronic diarrhea
10. Contusion
11. Endometriosis
12. Flaccid paralysis or paresis
13. Fracture and post-cast removal
14. Hernia
15. Joint instability/hypermobility
16. Kidney infection/stones
17. Mastitis
18. Minor surgery
19. Pelvic Inflammatory disease
20. Pitting edema
21. Portal hypertension
22. Prolonged constipation
23. Abortion/cesarean/vaginal birth
24. Trigeminal neuralgia

Other Important Considerations

Can Massage spread cancer?

There is no clinical evidence that lymphatic massage or any other type of massage spreads cancer by increasing lymph flow. Likewise, there is no evidence that it does not.

- Know when to consult with a medical Doctor and other health professionals.
- Emotional or Psychiatric conditions – Individual decision to have a session
- Some medications may affect touch sensitivity or thinning of the skin
- Allergies to certain oils/creams, cleansers/disinfectants
- Body – pins, staples, and artificial joints may alter the session

Refusal to Massage

A CLIENT MAY REFUSE A MASSAGE AT ANY TIME!

You will refuse to massage anyone with a fixed contra-indication or any flexible contra-indication you feel warrants it.

Simply advise the client that massage cannot be provided without a physician's written approval.

Under no circumstances can a client force you to provide a massage if you feel it is unsafe.

- Never massage a client with a fever!
- Fixed contra-indication!
- And if a pregnant client has pitted edema!

Client/Practitioner Boundaries

- Client Neglect
  - Unintentional physical or emotional harm resulting from practitioner insensitivity or lack of knowledge.
- Client Abuse
  - Physical or emotional harm sustained from deliberate acts of the practitioner
- Boundaries are best established and maintained through communication
- Confidentiality is a must with the client's session or written information. Please do not talk to anyone other than the client about their session. Unless the client has given a written release form. Other than being subpoenaed by court order.
- Client safety is a must! Physically and Emotionally
- Intellectual boundaries
  - Beliefs, thoughts, and ideas
- Financial boundaries
  - The price of a session will always be told and agreed upon before a session.
- A mistake many practitioners make is becoming a friend with the client. Business should stay business, and if a friendship develops outside of the massage room, then have the new friend go to someone else.
- If an intimate relationship should develop, it is said that six months of discontinuing the client-practitioner relationship before the new relationship is initiated.
- Even flirting is considered sexual misconduct and is not permitted.
- Selling products to a client is a conflict of interest. If you have products, they may be displayed outside the massage room and never be implied they must buy, only suggested they could buy. It

should be similar to a store, where a client may browse and look but not need to purchase anything else.

What Comes Next?

The factors that need to be considered when providing a massage include:
- Direction
- Pressure
- Rate and Rhythm
- Media
- Position and Client
- Duration
- Frequency

Direction

The overall directions of the massage strokes taught in the course are generally in the direction of the heart. However, lymph does not move in a direct line, so some guidelines are required. They will be stressed during practical massage periods; however, the movements are generally as follows:

- In the direction of the heart. This means from the toes and fingers in the direction towards the body. On the trunk, all movement should push the lymph toward the heart.

- In the direction of lymph flow. The lymph flows toward the heart; however, at times, it flows through its capillaries into lymph nodes that require movement other than toward the heart. The direction of massage is always toward these locations.

Pressure

First, it must be understood that pressure does not necessarily mean depth. To use more pressure does not mean working deeply. It means a greater weight on and during the stroke. The massage taught does not require hard pressure; however, often, the client has been told it is not a good massage without heavy pressure. Those clients need re-education. The lymph drainage massage used is very effective with light to moderate pressure.

The pressure must be adjusted to the client's condition and preferences. For example, more muscular clients may need heavier pressure to feel the stokes. This may not be important for effectiveness but may impact their mental and emotional needs.

The pressure of the stroke also should not depend upon muscular strength. If the stroke pressure is based on strength, the practitioner will tire after the massage. The pressure should be mostly derived through body weight and posture.

Grading of Touch

Grade 1-3   European Lymph Drainage or Hot Stone

Grade 4-6   Swedish Massage

Grade 7-8   Trigger Point or Table Shiatsu

Grade 9-10   Deep Tissue and Rolfing

Rate and Rhythm

Rate related to the number of strokes per minute.
Rhythm refers to the flow and routine.

The rate can create entirely different feelings and results
in a massage. A fast rate will invigorate, while a slow rate
tends to relax. Generally, a client should leave the
massage feeling relaxed and content. Therefore, the rate
should be slow, perhaps at about one per two inches per
second.

Rhythm is essential to a good massage. The biggest
mistake is to vary the rate and lose rhythm. Instead, all
movements should be at the same speed, and pause
between moves equal to the rhythm.

The basic rules are:

- The movement must be slow, gentle, and
  rhythmic.
- There must be no hesitancy, irregularity, or pauses
  in the movements.
- The time between the ending of the stroke and the
  start of the next one should be identical to the time
  of the stroking throughout the movement.

Media

The use of tools in massage for aromatherapy purposes is discouraged. It takes away the intimacy and awareness of the client's body. The only recommended tools are carrier oils and essential oils.

Position and Client

The client should be in a comfortable position. The preferred position for a full body massage is horizontal, with the face in a face cradle or resting while lying face down. However, the position will be dictated by the client's health and ability to assume the position. One example is a pregnant woman who cannot lie on her stomach.

The position of the therapist must be one of comfort. There should be no strain to reach any part of the client's body, and all moves should protect the therapist's lower back.

Duration

Some practitioners provide their clients with one and one-half hours or more massage. They believe they are providing excellent service for the money paid. If they are doing the massage for that duration for that reason, then it is between them and their client. Various experts have written on the subject dating back to Galen.

Although they all expressed differing times for the whole process, only one recommended a massage longer than 60 minutes. A therapist named, Mennell said the maximum should be 75 for neurasthenia, and only in a few cases.

Most limited the time on any area to about a maximum 4-10 minutes, with the majority agreeing that 40-50 minutes and, at the most, massages be between 50 and 60 minutes and that you vary the time according to the health and state of the client.

Frequency

The experts vary in the frequency they recommend for providing massage. Certainly, a daily massage in the method taught would not harm anyone and would likely be very beneficial.

However, the decision on frequency depends more on the client than the therapist. What their condition and finances allow must be considered. Even if a person is willing to spend money for a daily massage, you must consider the ethics and determine the benefit before obliging.

Basic Anatomy and Physiology - Specifically for Relaxation Massage

Swedish Massage works on and affects every system in the body. How Swedish Massage affects each system by a massage.

Cardiovascular System (Blood Circulation)
It consists of Heart, Blood, and Blood vessels (arteries, veins, and capillaries)

Function:
- Delivers oxygen and nutrients to the cells
- While carrying waste products away from the cells
- It helps maintain the acid-base balance in the body
- Protects against disease
- And helps regulate body temperature
- Combat Hemorrhage – clotting mechanisms

How massage affects the Cardiovascular system:
Massage can increase or decrease blood pressure and increase or decrease circulation to the body.

Digestive System (Food and Elimination)
Consists of: Gastro-intestinal tract; associated organs: mouth, stomach, pancreas, liver, gall bladder, small and large colon/intestine, and salivary glands

Function:
- Ingestion and digestion of food
- Absorption - physical and chemical breakdown of food into useable nutrients for the cells
- Defecation - Helps eliminate waste from the body

How massage affects the Digestive system:
Can be stimulated or depressed through massage

Endocrine System (Hormones)
Consists of: Hormone producing glands: Hypothalamus, Pituitary, Pineal, Thyroid, Parathyroid, Thymus, Adrenals, Pancreas, and Testes and Ovaries

Function:
- Regulates the body's activities through hormones and chemicals in the blood
- Produces and secretes hormones
- It assists the body in relaxing in times of stress
- Contributes to the reproductive process

How massage affects the Endocrine system:
Massage can stimulate or depress the number of hormones circulating through the body.

Immune System (Protection from invading pathogens)
Consists of: Works with the Lymphatic system and Organs (tonsils and appendix). The immune system tells the rest of the body how to defend itself.

Function:
- Destroy and eliminate pathogens, foreign substances, or toxic materials
- Non-specific Immunity
- Consists of: Skin, mouth, stomach, intestines, genitourinary tract, respiratory tract, eyes, and ears.
- Cellular response -Epithelium (skin and mucus), phagocytic (neutrophils, macrophages), and natural killer cells.
- Fever
- Inflammatory responses –Swelling, heat, a loss of function, redness, pain (vasodilation)
- Blood clotting
- Specific Immunity
- T- cells and B cells (help from the lymphatic system) activate if:

- o Pathogen travels to a lymph node
- o Pathogen travels to the spleen
- o Pathogen penetrates mucous membranes and comes in contact with embedded lymphatic nodules.
- Vaccinations can stimulate a response (build up resistance)

How massage affects the Immune system:
Massage helps to relax a person, and thus the body can work more efficiently. Light effleurage helps pump the lymphatic fluid through the body to help destroy invaders the immune system wants to destroy.

Integumentary System (Skin)
It consists of Skin, Hair, Nails, and Sweat or Oil Glands
Function:
- It helps regulate body temperature
- Protects body
- Immunity
- Absorption
- Eliminates some waste products
- Assists in the production of Vitamin D
- Sensation and receives stimuli like pressure, pain, and temperature

How massage affects the Integumentary system:
The massage takes place entirely on the skin's surface and so directly affects it. The skin contains sensors for pressure, temperature, and movement. It can be affected by the oils (carrier and aromatherapy) we use or how we hold our hands on its surface. The skin can be one of the first reactions to the massage that we see and can tell us a great deal about the person.

Lymphatic System (Eliminate waste and protection from invading pathogens)

It consists of Lymph, Lymphatic vessels, and Organs

Function:
- Transport- Returns proteins and plasma to the cardiovascular system and fats.
- Filters body fluid
- Produces white blood cells (T-cells)
- Immune response - protects the body from disease
- Eliminates some waste products
- Maintains homeostasis

How massage affects the Lymphatic system:
Light effleurage helps pump lymphatic fluid through the body. The Lymphatic system has no pump mechanism, so it needs motion to aid in the process of massage or exercise.

Muscular System (Muscles)

It consists of Connective tissue – Muscles, Fascia, and Heart organ

Function:
- Skeletal muscles
- Contract and move bones (joints: shoulder, elbow, wrist, fingers, neck, spine, ribs, hip, knee, ankle, and toes)
- Posture maintenance
- Heat production
- Movement helps lymph and blood flow
- Smooth muscles make up the heart organ

How massage affects the Skeletal-Muscular system:
Promotes or depresses muscle tone, fibers can relax,

Nervous System (Nerves)

It consists of Brain, Spinal Cord, Nerves, Cerebrospinal fluid, Neurotransmitters, and special sense organs such as eyes and ears.

Function:
- Sensory input and motor output
- Higher mental functioning and emotional responsiveness
- Regulates Body activity through nerve impulses
- Detects internal and external changes and stimuli
- Responding to those stimuli by inducing muscular contractions or glandular secretions

How massage affects the Nervous system:
The nervous system senses the stimulation from the massage (touch, pressure, rhythm, etc. and responds accordingly.

Reproductive System (Sexx organs)

It consists of Organs (testes, ovaries, prostate, uterus), ducts, and tubes that produce, store, and transport reproductive cells.

Function:
- Reproduction of that organism
- Produce offspring
- Release Hormones

How massage affects the Reproductive system:
Massage can be physically stimulated or aroused, or stimulated to increase the production of reproductive cells. Relaxation helps the body from fidgety.

Respiratory System (Breathing)
It consists of the Lungs and associated pathways, nose, pharynx

Function:
- Exchange of gases - Supplies oxygen and Eliminates carbon dioxide
- Olfaction (smell)
- Assists in regulating acid-base balance (homeostasis)
- Provides vocal sounds

How massage affects the Respiratory system:
Massage can promote deeper breathing, open airways, and relax muscles surrounding the lungs, enabling them to fill more effectively.

Skeletal System (Bones)
It consists of 206 bones, joints, cartilage, and ligaments

Function:
- Support
- Protection
- Movement
- Blood cell production
- Fat storage
- Mineral storage

How massage affects the Urinary system:
Improves joint mobility (ROM), alignment through muscle relaxation

Urinary System (Elimination)
It consists of the Kidneys, Ureters, Urethra, and Urinary bladder

Function:
- Regulate the chemical composition of blood, fluid, and electrolyte balance
- Assists in the elimination of wastes
- Red blood cell production
- Regulates blood pH
- Regulates blood pressure
- Maintains Homeostasis

How massage affects the Urinary system:
More or less waste is eliminated through stimulation of the organs and increasing or decreasing blood circulation, and organ function more efficiently.

Muscle Chart

Muscles (organs/meridian)

Organ/Meridian	Muscle
Ren/Central	Supraspinatus
Du/Governing	Teres major
Stomach	Pectoralis Major Clavicular
Spleen	Latissimus Dorsi
Heart	Subscapularis
Sm. Intestine	Quadriceps
Bladder	Peroneus
Kidney	Psoas
Paricardium/Cir/Sex	Gluteous Medius
Sanjiao/Triple Warmer	Teres Minor
Gall Bladder	Anterior Deltoid
Liver	Pectoralis Major Sternal
Lung	Anterior Serratus
Lg. Intestine	Fascia Lata

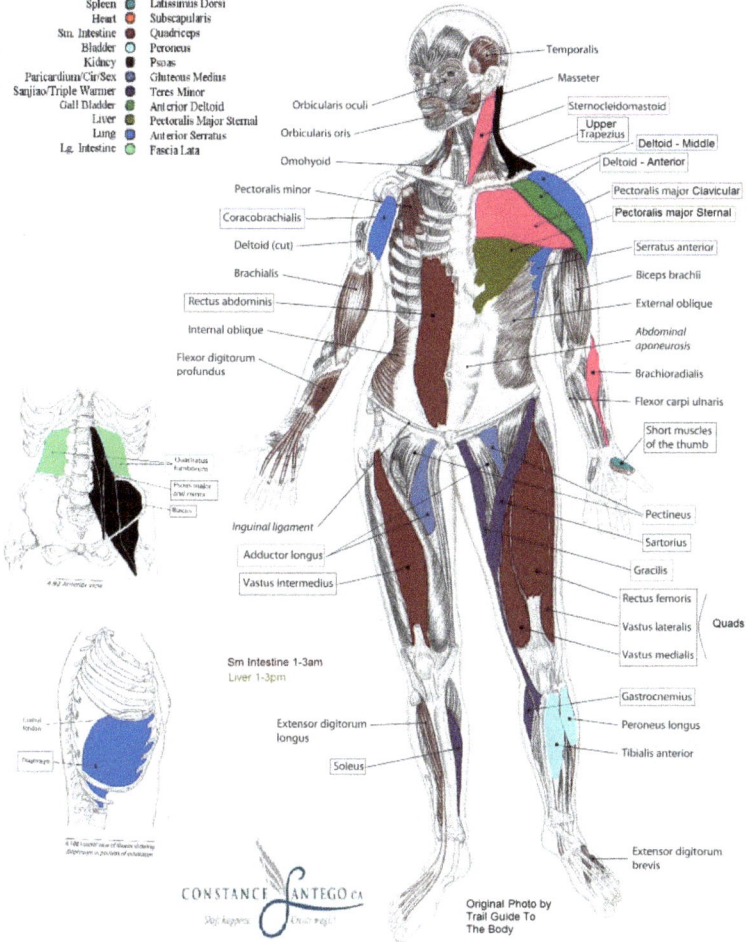

Temporalis
Masseter
Sternocleidomastoid
Upper Trapezius
Deltoid - Middle
Deltoid - Anterior
Pectoralis major Clavicular
Pectoralis major Sternal
Serratus anterior
Biceps brachii
External oblique
Abdominal aponeurosis
Brachioradialis
Flexor carpi ulnaris
Short muscles of the thumb
Pectineus
Sartorius
Gracilis
Rectus femoris
Vastus lateralis
Vastus medialis
Quads
Gastrocnemius
Peroneus longus
Tibialis anterior
Extensor digitorum brevis

Orbicularis oculi
Orbicularis oris
Omohyoid
Pectoralis minor
Coracobrachialis
Deltoid (cut)
Brachialis
Rectus abdominis
Internal oblique
Flexor digitorum profundus
Inguinal ligament
Adductor longus
Vastus intermedius
Extensor digitorum longus
Soleus

Sm Intestine 1-3am
Liver 1-3pm

CONSTANCE ANTEGO.ca

Original Photo by
Trail Guide To
The Body

Muscles (organs/meridians)

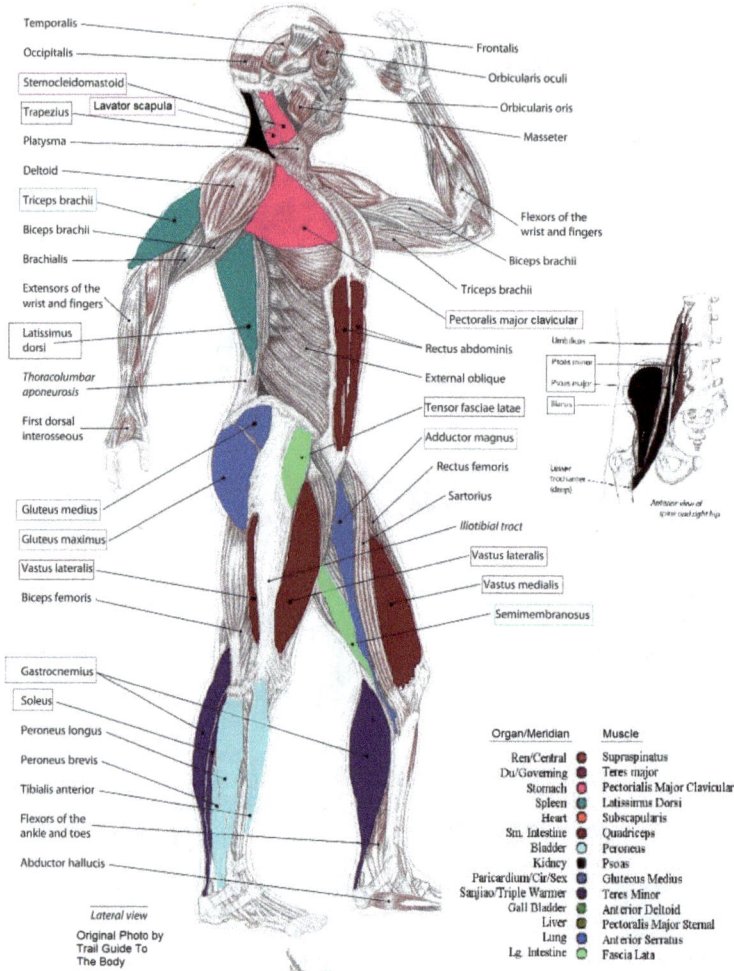

Temporalis
Occipitalis
Sternocleidomastoid
Trapezius — Lavator scapula
Platysma
Deltoid
Triceps brachii
Biceps brachii
Brachialis
Extensors of the wrist and fingers
Latissimus dorsi
Thoracolumbar aponeurosis
First dorsal interosseous
Gluteus medius
Gluteus maximus
Vastus lateralis
Biceps femoris
Gastrocnemius
Soleus
Peroneus longus
Peroneus brevis
Tibialis anterior
Flexors of the ankle and toes
Abductor hallucis

Frontalis
Orbicularis oculi
Orbicularis oris
Masseter
Flexors of the wrist and fingers
Biceps brachii
Triceps brachii
Pectoralis major clavicular
Rectus abdominis
External oblique
Tensor fasciae latae
Adductor magnus
Rectus femoris
Sartorius
Iliotibial tract
Vastus lateralis
Vastus medialis
Semimembranosus

Umbilicus
Psoas minor
Psoas major
Iliacus
Lesser trochanter (deep)
Anterior view of spine and right hip

Lateral view
Original Photo by Trail Guide To The Body

Organ/Meridian		Muscle
Ren/Central	●	Supraspinatus
Du/Governing	●	Teres major
Stomach	●	Pectoralis Major Clavicular
Spleen	●	Latissimus Dorsi
Heart	●	Subscapularis
Sm. Intestine	●	Quadriceps
Bladder	○	Peroneus
Kidney	●	Psoas
Paricardium/Cir/Sex	●	Gluteous Medius
Sanjiao/Triple Warmer	●	Teres Minor
Gall Bladder	●	Anterior Deltoid
Liver	●	Pectoralis Major Sternal
Lung	●	Anterior Serratus
Lg. Intestine	●	Fascia Lata

CONSTANCE SANTEGO.ca

Muscles (organs/meridians)

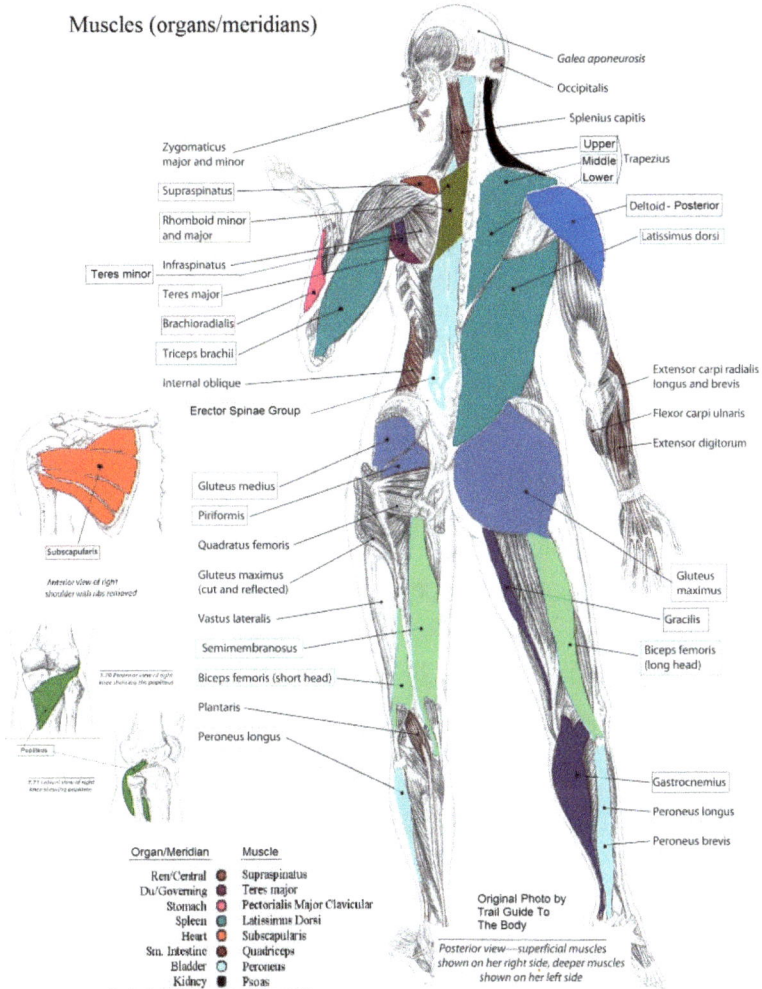

Galea aponeurosis
Occipitalis
Splenius capitis

Upper
Middle } Trapezius
Lower

Zygomaticus major and minor
Supraspinatus
Rhomboid minor and major
Infraspinatus
Teres minor
Teres major
Brachioradialis
Triceps brachii
internal oblique
Erector Spinae Group

Deltoid - Posterior
Latissimus dorsi

Extensor carpi radialis longus and brevis
Flexor carpi ulnaris
Extensor digitorum

Subscapularis
Anterior view of right shoulder with ribs removed

Gluteus medius
Piriformis
Quadratus femoris
Gluteus maximus (cut and reflected)
Vastus lateralis
Semimembranosus
Biceps femoris (short head)
Plantaris
Peroneus longus

Gluteus maximus
Gracilis
Biceps femoris (long head)

Gastrocnemius
Peroneus longus
Peroneus brevis

Popliteus

Original Photo by
Trail Guide To
The Body

Posterior view—superficial muscles shown on her right side, deeper muscles shown on her left side

Organ/Meridian		Muscle
Ren/Central		Supraspinatus
Du/Governing		Teres major
Stomach		Pectorialis Major Clavicular
Spleen		Latissimus Dorsi
Heart		Subscapularis
Sm. Intestine		Quadriceps
Bladder		Peroneus
Kidney		Psoas
Puricardium/Cir/Sex		Gluteus Medius
Sanjiao/Triple Warmer		Teres Minor
Gall Bladder		Anterior Deltoid
Liver		Pectoralis Major Sternal
Lung		Anterior Serratus
Lg. Intestine		Fascia Lata

Origin to Insertion

Skeletal muscles attach to bones through dense connective tissue called tendons. When injured (strain or tear), tendons will repair themselves over time, as they, unlike ligaments, have a blood supply. All muscles have an Origin and Insertion point or points. Muscles originate on a fixed bone and insert on a moveable bone. When a muscle contracts, the insertion point moves toward the origin.

Example:

The Biceps brachii

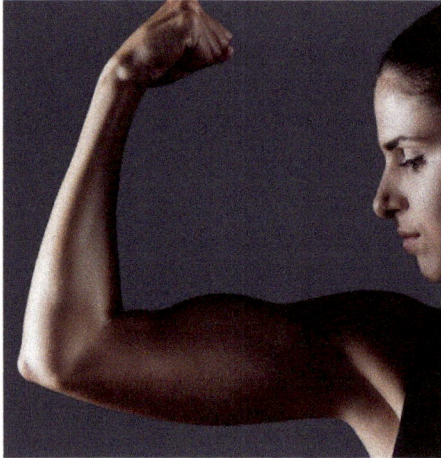

The Biceps brachii muscle in the arm originates at the scapula (supraglenoid tubercle of the scapula and the coracoid process). It inserts on the radius bone in the forearm (aponeurosis of the Biceps brachii and tubercle of radius).

When the muscle contracts, it flexes the arm at the elbow, moving the radius toward the scapula (shoulder).

Contraction

The main purpose of a muscle is to contract. The main muscle that creates the contraction is called the Agonist/Prime Mover. The one that opposes this action is the Antagonist. Synergist muscles help the agonist in action, and Fixators stabilize the joints in a given position so that the agonist can exert its action.

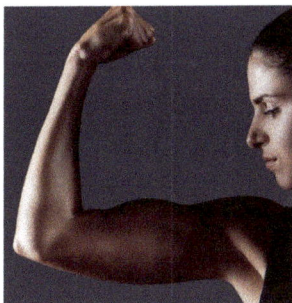

Example: **Agonist (Contracting / Shortening)**
Biceps brachii would be the agonist when the forearm is flexed towards the shoulder.

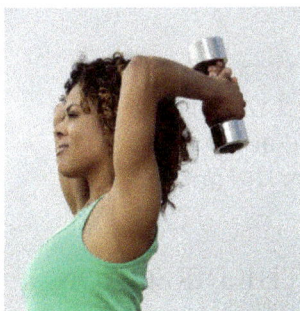

Antagonist (Relaxing / Lengthening)
Triceps brachii would be the Antagonist when the forearm is flexed towards the shoulder.

***Reversed when the arm is being extended. *Triceps Brachii would be the agonist, and Biceps Brachii would be the antagonist.*
Synergist (Helps move) - would be the Pronator teres,
Fixator (Stabilizes shoulder) - would be the Deltoids

Fiber Direction

All muscles have one or more fiber direction(s), depending on the type of muscle. The muscle fiber direction is always towards the origin.

Examples: As in the muscle shown previously - Biceps brachii, there are two directions (Bi). Triceps brachii has three (Tri).

Hint: Most origin muscle fiber direction is usually towards the heart. The neck has many that go in both directions, towards and away. If you are doing relaxation massage, create your moves to use pressure towards the heart and no pressure on the return.

Some muscles twist as they contract, as in Levator Scapula and Latissimus Dorsi, to name a couple.

Just Remember!!!

- o   Muscle always moves toward the origin
- o   Muscle always moves a bone at a joint
- o   Muscle contraction is always the action

TO BE SAFE: MASSAGE IN THE DIRECTION
OF THE HEART

Fascia

Fascia is a solid connective tissue surrounding muscles and bones and providing structural support.

Some of the best information you will find is in Luigi Stecco's book, *Fascial Manipulation for Musculoskeletal Pain.*

Massage Therapists focus a lot of attention on Superficial and Deep Fascia.

Superficial fascia is comprised of subcutaneous loose connective tissues containing a web of collagen, as well as primarily elastic fibers. It acts as both a mechanical and thermal cushion and facilitates the gliding of the skin above the deep fascia. SF contains fat, or fascicule of muscular tissue, and cutaneous vessels and nerves.

Deep Fascia is formed by a connective membrane that sheaths all muscles. The deep fascia, devoid of fat, forms sheaths for the nerves and vessels, becomes specialized around the joints to form or strengthen ligaments, envelops various organs and glands, and binds all of the structures together into a firm, compact mass.

- Working the fascia will create more space between the skin and muscle fibers for water to get to the area needed for protein to get to the cells, which is necessary for healing.
- It will take the normal eighteen days to two years to heal the fascia.
- If a bruise is created in a muscle, the fascia is like a sponge and will soak up the liquid but need manual drainage to release it.

- Will run in lengths throughout the body - hip to shoulder. So, it would be best if you worked the whole area to have a release happen.
- Old damaged injuries will have fascia holding the position. Release the fascia to balance the alignment of the person.

Anatomical Position

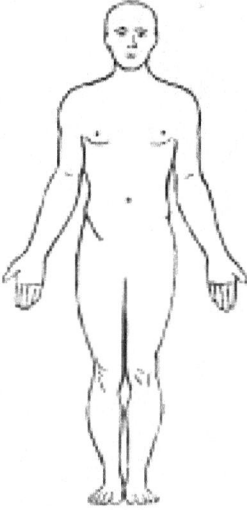

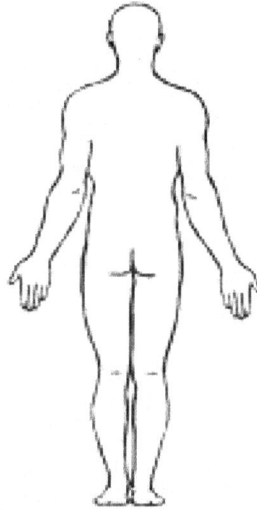

Anterior   Posterior

Anterior
- The position of the human body, standing erect, with the face directed anteriorly, the upper limbs at the sides and the palms turned anteriorly (supinated), and the feet pointed anteriorly.

Posterior
- Opposite

Movements of the Body

Motion	Opposite
• Extension	Flexion
• Adduction	Abduction
• Medial Rotation	Lateral Rotation
• Elevation	Depression
• Supination	Pronation
• Inversion	Eversion
• Plantar flexion	Dorsiflexion
• Protraction	Retraction

- Lateral Flexion of the neck
- Circumduction of the hip or shoulder
- Rotation of the spine
- Deviation of the mandible
- The opposition of the thumb (when it crosses the palm toward the pinkie)

Body Mechanics/Ergonomics

In massage therapy, how you position your body during a massage must have a direct relationship with the effectiveness of your massage.

Balance, breathing, strength, and stability are all essential to body mechanics to reduce the risk of an injury to your own body.

Table Height, when you stand by the table, your knuckles should glide just over the top. If it is too high, your shoulders will be elevated, and you will injure yourself. If it is too low, you may hurt your back by "hunching over" the client.

Height may need to be adjusted to the girth of your client. Some people have bigger bodies than others, and their tummies make them higher than you are used to. You may need to work with the height you have it at for the first massage and make a note for future massages. *If you have a hydraulic table, you can adjust it while the client is on the table.*

Body Stances

You will use your whole body to massage, NOT just your hands and arms. Meaning: when doing a massage technique, your body should move with your arms. If you use your whole body, you will not tire as quickly.

Get behind your work - stand behind the motion and flow forward.

The two main stances you will use while massaging a client are the Bow (Archer) and Horse (Warrior) stances.

Bow Stance
It is used when applying massage techniques that proceed from one point to the next along the client's body (effleurage).

- Your weight is mainly on your back leg while your front foot stabilizes (30° to 50° angle).

- Keep most of your weight on your back leg, using your front leg for balance.

- Lounge position,

- Knees slightly bent,

- The back is straight.

- One foot is facing straight forward (leading foot), and the other is pointing in the direction the therapist's body is moving (trailing foot).

- Your whole body follows the direction of the leading foot.

- Bend at the hips and knees as you lounge forward. Your arms should be extended perpendicular to your body but not locked.

- As you do compression movements, use your weight and leverage to "lean" – not your muscles to "push" – on your client.

Horse Stance

It is used when applying massage techniques that traverse (travel) relatively short distances (pétrissage and friction).

- The feet are facing the same direction, towards the table side, and the knees are slightly bent.
- The back is straight, and the pelvis is tilted posteriorly (tummy in, groin out).
- Relax your shoulders while your hands and arms are moving.
- You may move up and down as needed by flexing your knees more.
- Also, you can move side to side by shifting from one gluteal muscle to the other (bum) as you move to the part of the client's body you are massaging.

The most stable base for the body is two feet on the ground, and in the triangle structure, two feet on the ground and your hands are on the client. Your lower body is 2 ½ times stronger than your upper body.

Summary of points to consider regarding Body Mechanics:

- Align your body and feet apart for stability. Knees relaxed. Most of your weight should be on your back foot, while the pressure you apply to your client will be mainly from the opposite hand.
- Stay behind the stroke. As you massage your client, be sure you are directing the stroke. You should be able to maintain an angle of 45° to 60° with your arms. If you are at 90°, you may injure your arms and shoulders.
- Wrists and hands must always be relaxed. Tension is transmitted to the client through your hands, so you must also be comfortable to make them feel comfortable.
- Use your fingers and thumbs as little as possible. For Swedish massage, a broad open-palm contact will be more comfortable for your client and easier on your body.
- Keep your wrists flat. The greater the angle of your wrist, the better off you will be. Ideally, your wrist should never have an angle of less than 110°. A sharper angle than this could cause compression on the nerves in your wrist.
- Always face the client. This will help avoid twisting your body and pulling or straining your muscles.

Sitting down while massaging.

When working on the client's feet, hands, neck, shoulders, or face, you may sit down occasionally on a chair or an exercise ball. The suggestion is twenty-five percent of the time. Leaning your hip on the table may be used if in one area for a while.

Client Care

Sheets, Blankets, Bolsters, and Pillows are used for client comfort. Pillows and bolsters will be placed under the sheets. They must have a protective, washable cover if used over.

- All pressure and techniques are to the client's tolerance.
- It is best to have a bolster, half bolster, or pillow under the client's ankles while in the prone position (face down). This will support and maintain proper body alignment of the client's joints and help the muscle relax.
- It is best to have bolsters, half bolsters, or a pillow under the client's knees while in the supine position (face-up). This will reduce tension in the hips and lower back.
- They may require a pillow under their tummy while prone.
- Some clients need a small rolled-up towel under their neck while supine
- Some clients need a small rolled-up towel under their upper chest to relieve the breast area while prone.
- Pregnant clients or the elderly may be the best side-lying with pillows under their head, between their legs, and by their tummy.
  - (Pregnant clients, if lying on their back, would need pillows under their head, many pillows under their knees, and one <u>under</u> the right side of the tummy (*to keep the pressure off of their main blood artery*)
- Some clients like a semi-reclining position. Many pillows may be used under their back and head to lift them into a 40° or 45° angle.

- Clean sheets and face covers are always used per client — top and bottom (single or twin should fit your massage table). A blanket can be used as a need for the client to stay warm. When a client is being massaged, they will go into a state of relaxation/meditation while lower their body temperature.

CLEANING

Hygiene is very, very important!!!
- Cross-contamination
    - Hands are the number one source of cross-contamination!
    - Have a pump for the oil.

Draping/Toweling

You will put:

- A sheet under the client
- A sheet on top (unless you have been taught the toweling technique).
- A face cover covering the head /face rest.
- A blanket over the top sheet (you will need to be able to wash these with each client)
- Pillows or bolsters as needed (cover with a case)
- A breast towel (large enough to cover large breasts)

For clients, comfort, and warmth, only one area should be uncovered.

Your Mood

Your Body Language will affect how the client will enjoy the massage. For example, the client will know if you are angry, upset, mad, happy, or sad!

Try this, have a person sit on a chair backward, so their back is facing you. You can give them a pillow to lean on. Ask them to tell you what they feel.

- First, massage their back for a few moments.
- Now, have an intent of being happy, massage their back for a few moments. Then, ask them what they felt.
- Now, have an intent of being sad, massage their back for a few moments. Ask them what they felt.
- Now, have an intent of being in love, massage their back for a few moments. Ask them what they felt.
- Now, have an intent of being angry, massage their back for a few moments. Then, ask them what they felt.
- Now, if you want ice cream, massage their back for a few moments. Ask them what they felt.

You get the idea. As you change your intent, the pressure and rhythm of your movements change.

Massage Oil

You can use cream, but most practitioners use oil. The two most popular oils to use are Grapeseed Oil and Olive Oil. Both have an excellent glide to them when you massage.

Grapeseed Oil - *Vitis vinifera*

- Source: Seed
- Odor: None
- Contra-indications: None - Hypoallergenic
- Color: Pale Green
- Feel: Satin Like
- Shelf life: 2 years
- Blending ability: 100%

Helps -   Skin: Acne, slightly astringent, tones, tightens, and maintains firmness and elasticity.

Olive Oil - *Olea europaea*

- Source: Fruit
- Odor: Strong
- Contra-indications: None - Hypoallergenic
- Color: Pale Yellow - Greenish
- Feel: Normal
- Shelf life: 2 years
- Blending ability: Best at 10-50% but can be 100%

Helps -   Skeletal: Arthritis and Rheumatism

Muscular: Sprains and Bruises

Coconut Oil - *Cocos nucifera*

60/40 Fractionated 100%

- Source: Coconut Kernel
- Odor: Strong
- Contra-indications: May be an allergy reaction
- Color: Clear
- Feel: Greasy
- Shelf life: 2 years
- Blending ability: 10%

Helps -   Skin: Emollient, Suntanning

Jojoba Oil - *Simmondsia chinensis*

- Source: Seed
- Odor: Light
- Contra-indications: None - Hypoallergenic
- Color: Clear
- Feel: Normal
- Shelf life: 2 years
- Blending ability: 100%

Helps -   Skeletal: Arthritis and Rheumatism

Skin: Dry, Skin infections, Scalp disorders, some sunscreen properties, BUT, it can clog pores.

Anti-inflammatory

Castor Oil - *Ricinus communis*

- Source: Seed
- Odor: None
- Contra-indications: None
- Color: Clear
- Feel: Thick
- Shelf life: 2 Years
- Blending ability: 10%

Helps -   Skin: Emollient, Suntanning

CASTOR OIL PACK:

For Pain Reduction and to break-up Scar Tissue, Stretch Marks, Moles, Warts, and Endometriosis

Blending ability: 100%

Castor oil is multi-purpose vegetable oil. It's made by extracting oil from the seeds of the *Ricinus communis* plant. Castor oil is a particular type of triglyceride fatty acid; nearly 90 percent of its fatty acid substance is ricinoleic acid, an unsaturated omega-9 fatty acid.

In History, castor oil was burned as fuel in lamps, used as a natural remedy to treat ailments like eye irritation, and even given to pregnant women to stimulate labor. Castor oil remains a popular natural treatment for common conditions like constipation and skin ailments. It is commonly used in natural beauty products.

Castor oil has no noted interactions with other drugs.

This oil is known to be a powerful laxative (*rinconelic acid in castor oil can help relieve occasional constipation*), **support the immune system, is a natural moisturizer, promotes wound healing, acne reduction, fights fungus (such as warts or candida), keep hair and scalp healthy, and is easily absorbed by the tissue being treated.** In addition, applying castor oil packs to any body parts trauma, such as sprains, bruises, or tissue build-up, will help relieve pain, reduce spasms, and benefit the healing process by minimizing swelling and relaxing the injured area.

Castor Oil is best known for its *lymph-stimulating abilities and its anti-inflammatory qualities*. As the oil is absorbed into the body, its vibratory action stimulates the parasympathetic nerves located in the area, activating the lymphatic system to drain. This process benefits and organ(s) or body part with restricted circulation flow. By increasing the movement of lymph through the vessels, this oil is one of the most effective agents for stimulating muscular and mucous membrane activity.

The digestive and nervous systems also have a primary effect when castor oil is used. Castor oil helps to coordinate the activity between the functions of the organs. An example is to help cleanse the gall bladder and liver of toxins.

CONTRA-INDICATIONS

- **Do not apply to open wounds.**
- Castor oil can cause side effects, such as **allergic reactions and diarrhea**, in some people.
- Avoid use if hypersensitivity, GI obstruction or perforation, severe impaction, symptoms of appendicitis or acute surgical abdomen, ulcerative colitis, and rectal fissures.
- It can also induce labor, **so pregnant women should avoid it.**

TOPICAL USES FOR CASTOR OIL

- Arthritis Treatment
- To Strengthen and Grow Hair
- Acne Treatment
- Skin Moisturizer
- Deep Cleanser
- To Improve Immunity Function
- To Eliminate Fine Lines and Wrinkles
- Reduce Swelling and Inflammation
- Support Lymphatic System
- Increase Circulation
- Heal Wounds and Abrasions

- Relieve Menstrual Cramps

ORAL USES FOR CASTOR OIL

- Relieve Constipation
- Clean Out Intestines Before Surgery
- Induction of Labor

APPLICATIONS:

Apply it to the skin as a massage oil, use it through a castor oil pack, or mix it with other oils as a topical remedy. Orally, add it to milk or lukewarm water or take it as a supplement. It is an old remedy to take a tablespoon of castor oil to cleanse the colon *(make sure to do it first thing in the morning before eating - it moves everything fast)*. Talk to your health provider before trying internally.

CASTOR OIL PACK PROCEDURE:

My favorite.

NEEDED FOR CASTOR OIL PACK:

- Castor Oil
- Cotton pad/cloth (white)
- Saran Wrap

Step #1: Clean the area to place the pack

Step #2: Using unbleached cotton flannel fabric, fold the cotton cloth into a pad (three-four layers). You *can reuse the cotton pad for step 7 (new cotton pad needed for step 8) if using it for a short period of time (up to 15 - 45 minutes) put a heating pad or hot water bottle over the area.*

Step #3: Soak the pad with Castor Oil (not dripping, but all material covered and saturated – *add more oil each day)*

- Reuse the pads by placing them in a Ziploc bag in the refrigerator until you're ready to use them again.

Step #4: Place the soaked cotton pad over the area on the body related to the pain, trauma, or health issue.

Step #5: Using the Saran wrap, wrap it many times around the part of the body with the cotton pad, *not too tight.* This acts as a vapor barrier to hold the castor oil in.

Step #6: Minimum 45 minutes, but **best to sleep overnight with the pad on** - 8 - 12 hours (*if using while sleeping, use old sheets and nightwear – the oil may stain cloth)*

Step #7: Repeat (steps 1-6) for three (3) days, *best is; you know you are done with the daily application when you see oil floating in the toilet after urinating.*

Step #8: Repeat every 1 to 3 months - for three more times or until the pain/issue is relieved

Store oil in a protected container for future use.

Massage Table or Chair

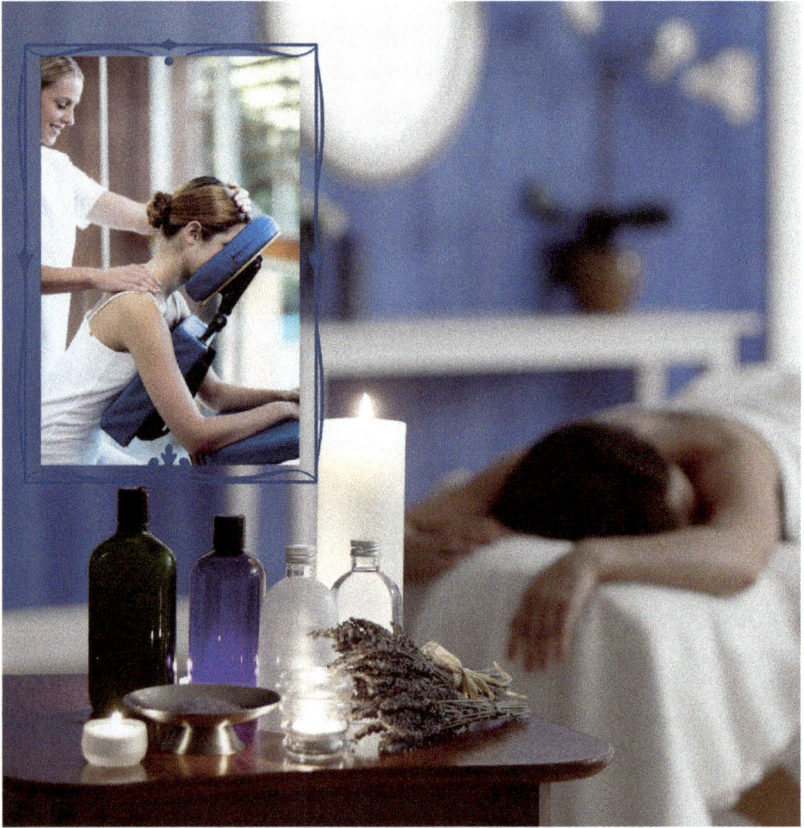

You can massage someone almost anywhere, but most professionals use a massage table or massage chair.

Portable Massage Table:

- Weight of the table; 30-40 pounds (14-18 kilograms)
- Usually made with a wood frame
- Length is 72 inches x 29 to 32 inches wide
- The 3-inch thickness of dense foam
- Heavy-duty vinyl upholstery
- Folds up
- It can be put into a bag for transporting from place to place. *I use this, and I leave it set up in my room.*
- Comes with a face rest. Some headrests are adjustable.
- It holds approximately 300 pounds
- $300 plus

Hydraulic tables – Not portable! Many Chiropractors and Physiotherapists use these types of tables.

- Similar in looks and upholstery
- Metal frame
- Stationary - Very heavy to move
- Electrical – The height of the table can easily be adjusted with a switch.
- Holds approximately 600 pounds
- $1000's

Sheets – you can purchase custom-sized sheets, but single/twin sizes will fit.

Face protector - you can purchase washable and disposable covers

Cover with a low-back heated bag, a cozy blanket, a sheepskin underlay, and relaxation.

Massage Chair – The client is facing forwards in a sitting position.

- Usually made with a wood frame
- Heavy-duty vinyl upholstery
- Folds up
- It can be put into a bag for transporting from place to place. *I use this, and I leave it set up in my room.*
- Comes with adjustable face rest and armrest.
- It holds approximately 265 pounds
- $300 plus

PART TWO

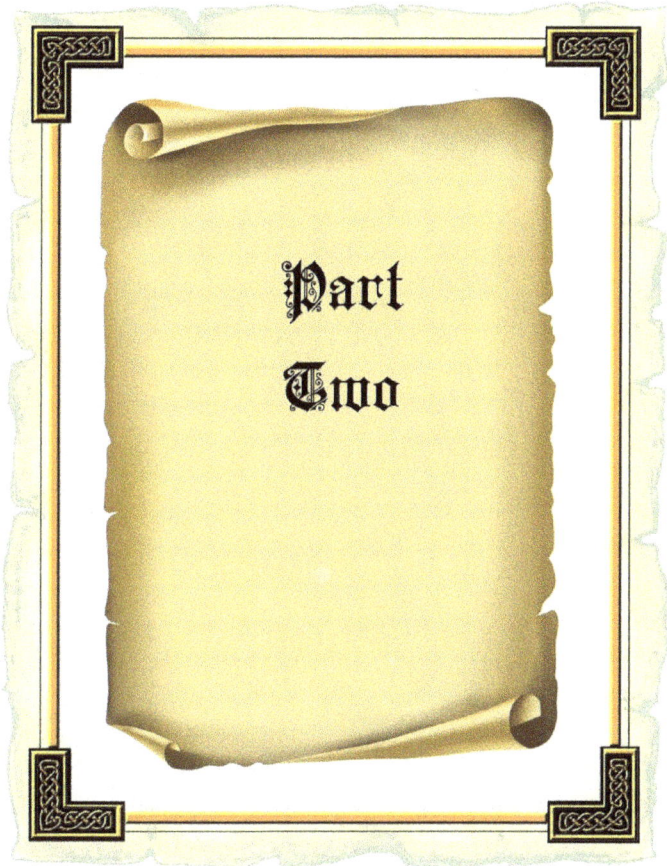

Setting up for the Massage

ake sure that your table is set to the correct height for you. If it is too high, having a footstool for the client to use when it is time to get on the table is a good idea.

Make sure you have two sheets (top and bottom) as well as 1 to 2 towels, a face rest cover, pillows or bolsters, and carrier oil or lotion you may be using. Having a blanket nearby or already on the table for extra warmth is a good idea.

Do your client consultation before they get undressed, so you can find their medical history and current status before they are on the table. This is the time to get to know your client. Find out their medical history. Do they have any contra-indications? How are they feeling today?

If you are a practitioner- REMEMBER to chart everything! If you see a sore or a bruise, record it! If a client tells you something hurts, record it! If a client falls asleep on the table, record it! Use chat and recordkeeping for your protection. It will also help you follow a client's progress from session to session. If in any doubt, RECORD IT!

Clearly explain what is to be expected of the client and what you will do, and find out what their expectation is of you. For example, if they require assistance in getting undressed, you can help them. Otherwise, explain that you are leaving the room and will return when they are on the table. Tell them what position you want them to begin with on the massage table.

General Rules to Massage

1. Superficial – Deep – Superficial
2. General – Specific – General
3. Proximal – Distal – Proximal
4. Movement (pressure) is in the direction of the heart, and lymphatic flow

Superficial (light) – Deep – Superficial (light): Tissue must always be warmed up before deep or specific moves can be performed. Therefore, the massage starts light, works into deeper pressure, and then returns to light.

General – Specific – General: Before working on a specific area in that region, you will always start to massage a larger area first to Warm-up that area (for example: all of the back or all of a leg).

Proximal – Distal – Proximal: (Usually means for the arms and legs) Generally, when you start, start close to the torso, move down the body, then back up the body to finish. Think of it as head to toe to head.

Basic Movements

Resting Position

It seems like a little thing, but this will set the mood and the effectiveness of the whole massage. The resting position is how and where you place your hands on the client's body before you begin massaging them, as well as your positioning between movements. This must be done with respect to a client's boundaries. A slow, steady approach is essential. Your touch should be confident but not hard. An open, soft, relaxed, warm, and dry hand is best. This will help your client to feel at ease with you. Remember – they are in a very vulnerable position, being naked or nearly naked on the table. You are clothed, standing over them. This is the first ultimate power position and must not be taken for granted. It is a good idea to first touch your client on the shoulder or between the shoulder blades. These are both reasonably non-threatening positions.

Effleurage
(Broad stroke)

Effleurage comes from the French verb meaning 'To skim' or 'To touch lightly on.' Effleurage begins lightly, but altering the stroke's pressure, speed, rhythm, and direction can be adapted to almost any situation. Effleurage is gliding along with the muscle in a horizontal direction with the muscle. The glide goes in the same general direction as the muscle. If applied slowly and steadily, it is a soothing and relaxing movement. When applied quickly, it is very stimulating or invigorating. Great for assessing, treating and re-assessing

- Long, Slow, gliding movements that are repeated
- Use for the beginning and end of each area
- Can use palm, finger, thumbs, fist, forearm, elbow *(knee or foot- as in Thia massage)*
  - One-Handed
    - Ironing, Circular (sun and moon)
  - Two-Handed
    - Heart (back, neck, and shoulders), Circular
  - Alternate Hands
    - Raking, Circular, Open C's
  - Nerve stroke
    - Feathering (with fingers)

Effects
- Relaxing when done slowly
- Stimulating and invigorating when done fast
- Increases skin temperature
- Increases blood flow
- Stimulates lymph flow
- Improves mobility of the skin and subcutaneous tissue
- Increase range of motion

- Client/Practitioner touch
  - Body contour, tissue quality, and other palpatory assessment
- The transition between massage techniques, smoother sequence, and continuity
- Promote movement of intestinal contents
- Promote absorption of inflammatory by-products in sub-acute and chronic stages of soft tissue injury.

Stroking
(Broad and Intermediate stroke)

Stroking is like Effleurage, but no return motion

Pétrissage
(Intermediate and Specific stroke)

Pétrissage is a different kind of movement; its directional focus is vertical to the muscle. Pétrissage is very good for decreasing muscle tone, as it "tricks" the muscle tissue into relaxing, by stimulating the pressure sensor receptors in the tendons.

- Kneading, lifting, rolling, squeezing, compressing, and releasing
- Milk the tissue of waste and draw new blood and oxygen
  - Can use: palm, finger, thumbs
  - One-Handed
    - Great for arms, forearms, or shoulders
- Two-Handed

- ▪ Praying hands, ocean waves, fulling (broadening)
  - Alternate Hands
    - ▪ Skin rolling

Effects

- Relaxing when done slowly
- Stimulating and invigorating when done fast
- Increases skin temperature
- Increases blood flow
- Increase range of motion
- Reduces muscle soreness and stiffness
- Promote absorption of inflammatory by-products in sub-acute and chronic stages of soft tissue injury.

Compression
(Intermediate stroke)

Compression is a non-gliding technique of sustained pressure or a sequence of alternating rhythmic pressures (To press together or squeeze).

- Fluid exchange
- Force applied at a 90° angle perpendicular to the muscle belly and a 45° angle along the spine or anterior leg.
  - o Can use palm, finger, thumbs, knuckles, fist, forearm, or elbow (knee or foot- as in Thia massage)
  - o One-Handed - Press – release 8 to 10 seconds
  - o Two-Handed (can be stacked)
  - o May use a rocking motion
- Effects
  - o Relaxing when done slowly
  - o Stimulating and invigorating when done fast

- o Increases blood flow (localized)
- o Increase range of motion

Friction
(Intermediate stroke)

The application direction is usually across the muscle fibers when using the friction movement. You may need to press down into the muscle tissue before fractioning, but this is an excellent method to release adhesions and tense muscles.

- To rub, rubbing one surface back and forth over another in several directions.
- Shearing force
- Use little or no oil
- Superficial
  - o Can use hands, palms, fingers, knuckles, or towel
  - o Superficial warming- heat rub, sawing/ironing (ulna), towel friction
  - o Rolling – move arm skin, back and forth (quickly), hold hands on opposite sides of the arm
  - o Wringing – compressed and slower back and forth. Hold same hands side
- Deep *next three are: 10 seconds across fiber, with fiber or around
  - o Cross fiber - using fingers – deep, transverse friction, perpendicular (to client's tolerance)
  - o Chucking - using fingers – parallel friction
  - o Circular – using fingers or palm – around in circles
- Effects
  - o Increases blood flow
  - o Stimulates lymph flow

- Promote absorption of inflammatory by-products in sub-acute and chronic stages of soft tissue injury.
- It may reduce posttraumatic scar tissue and adhesions (skin, muscle, tendons, ligaments, and joints
- Relieves pain and muscle spasms – promoting relaxation
- Produces localized vasodilatation (widening of blood vessels)

Vibration
(Intermediate and Specific stroke)

Vibration is an 'up and down' or 'side to side' movement on the muscles. It can be relatively 'coarse' or 'fine.' Vibration is perhaps one of the most difficult manipulations to master, and it takes practice to become proficient at it.

- Can use hands, fingers, or appliance
- Rapid to slow
- Quivering (very light touch, barely touching client)
- Trembling (just touching the client)
- Jostling / Shaking – relaxing large muscle groups (side to side direction)
  - Coarse (vigorous) vibration - no flow
  - Fluffing (lifting)
- Rocking – (full-body movement) rhythmic technique - flows

Effects

- Promotes Relaxation
- Stimulating and invigorating when done fast
- Loosens phlegm
- Promote movement of intestinal contents
- It may facilitate muscle contraction

Tapotement/Percussion
(Specific stroke)

This comes from the French verb 'to rap, drum, or pat.' Tapotement involves repetitive staccato striking movements of the hands, either simultaneously or alternately. The hands, or parts of the hands, administer springy blows to the client's body at a fast rate. This also takes practice to become proficient without beating on the client".

- Draining fluid from a cavity
- It can be used to end a massage area.
  - Can use the ulna side of the hand, tips or flats of fingers, open or closed cupped palm, or the knuckles.
  - Clapping – slapping, splatting (using a palmer surface), use very lightly when on the face. NEVER on the BUM
  - Cupping – (sound of a running horse hoof sound) Great for respiratory issues
  - Diffused – one relaxed outstretched <u>hand</u> on the client, the other hand (relaxed <u>fist</u>) strikes your relaxed hand.
  - Hacking (ulna) – Quaking (3 fingers) muscle relaxation
    - DO NOT USE ON FATIGUED (tired) MUSCLES
- Pincement – plucking (as if pulling a Kleenex from the box) - strike, grasp, lift, release
- Pounding (knuckles) / Beating (ulna side of the fist) beating or rapping
- Tapping – raindrops (fingers tap)

Athletic Massage

Massage

It is the manipulation of superficial and deeper layers of muscle and connective tissue to enhance function and promote relaxation and wellbeing.

Sports Massage

It was initially developed to help athletes prepare their bodies for optimal performance, recover after a big event, and function at top levels during training. In addition, sports massage emphasizes preventing and healing muscle and tendon injuries.

Athletic Massage Course

It intends to take the Swedish Massage techniques and provide a framework to apply them to each sport. As a result, you will give a great massage and help your client prepare for their activity by improving their performance and recovery time after an event.

The key difference is, with Athletic Massage, your intent will be working on specific muscles to increase mobility.

Although you will work on specific muscles with a more specific purpose, you will not assess or treat problems or injuries.

Again, you are **not** trying to **treat** anything with your client.

You can and should take note of anything you notice and refer your client for treatment (Medical Doctor, Massage Therapy, Physiotherapist, Chiropractor, etc.).

You are not preparing to treat these injuries, but knowing these are the problem areas helps you identify where you can most help. Preventative injury and muscle mobility

Contra-indications are the same as with Swedish Massage We will still be adhering to the basic rules and principles of Swedish Massage.

Baseball

Baseball is a full-body sport.

Baseball tends to have a large population of weekend warriors *(For example, non-athletic people in sports also tend to ignore warm-ups and stretches)*.

*The common problems most people playing baseball have is primarily in the shoulder and the knee.

Your focus will be on the hips, knees, and shoulders— some torso for the trunk rotation.

Massage Procedure: Prone position *(facing down)*

Upper Back

Do a routine Swedish massage

Lower Back

Starting at the Iliac crest (hip);

- Oil on
- Warm-up area (make sure it is ready for a bit deeper pressure)
- Do a deep palmar glide up towards the lower rib border – **3x** (start lighter and each time go a bit deeper)
- Supported fist glide/stripping just above iliac crest (hip) toward the outside of the hip – **3x**
- Beating/Pounding to the low back area and over the sheets on the glutes – **3x**

Hips

Through the sheet;

- Warm-up area
- Fist or elbow glide /stripping moving with the direction of the glutes from the top of the hip down to the upper hamstring. – **3x**
- **Repeat on the other side.**

Back of the Leg

- Oil on
- Warm-up area
- Supported fist friction with and crossed fiber to the upper hamstring (origin). – **6x** (3 in each direction)
- Deep palmar gliding up the hamstring – **9x** *(Separate into 3 sections, 3x each)*
- Fist glide/stripping along the outside aspect of the thigh – **3x** *(caution of depth, the I T band can be tender)*
- **Move to calf**

Back of the Calf

- Warm-up
- Deep thumb kneading over both heads of the calf. – **1x**
- Supported fist glide/stripping down both sides of the calf down to just above the Achilles tendon – **6x** *(3 per side, caution of the pressure used at the end of the stroke)*
- Deep palmar gliding at base of calf above

Achilles tendon – **4x**

- **Repeat the back of the leg on the other leg**

Front of the Legs-Quads

- Oil on
- Warm-up
- Deep palmar gliding (Starting at the upper sheet border) down the thigh to the knee – **5x** *(caution pressure around knee area)*
- Beating and pounding, making sure to do the full area.
- Thumb kneading around the kneecap *(Especially at the top area of the kneecap, this feels good).* - **X9** *(3 to the left, 3 to the center, 3 to the right)*
- **Repeat on the other leg.**

Front of the Calf

- Warm-up
- Supported elbow glide/stripping along the Tibial border and slightly more to the outside. – **4x**
- **Repeat on the other leg.**

Turn Over, Position: Face-up

Chest

- Oil on
- Warm-up
- Fingertip kneading-compressions to

upper chest – **4x**
- Fist glide/stripping from chest to shoulder – **3x**
- Fist glide /stripping edge of pecs and front of the shoulder *(with client arm out to side and hand raised -hello wave)* – **3x**

Arms

- Do the ELD arm routine
- **Repeat on the other arm**

Neck

- Oil on and Warm-up
- Fingertip gliding, both hands along both sides of the neck, from base to skull-**3x**
- Fist glide /stripping down the right side of the neck *(holding the client's head in your left hand)* – **3x**
- **Repeat on the other side**
- Fingertip is kneading the base of the skull.

Golf

This sport gives you an interesting mix of upper and lower body challenges.

Here you have to consider your client's tendencies:

A right-handed golfer will require a focus on the right chest and left shoulder (posterior deltoids). And with a left-handed athlete, focus on the left chest and right posterior deltoids.

*Low back injuries compete fairly evenly with Wrist, Forearm, and Shoulder injuries.

Your focus – Low Back, Upper back, Shoulders, Forearms, and Chest.

Upper and Lower Back

- Start with a routine Swedish massage
- Deep elbow glide/stripping from the Sacral border to above the lower ribs. – **3x** *(Caution crossing the lower rib border)*
- Deep glide/stripping along Thoracic Spine in 2 sections, - **6x** *(3 each)*
- Raking with fingertips along the ribs – **9x-12x** *(3-4 positions up ribs)*
- Deep hand glide (stripping) along the spinal border of the scapula. *(moving strokes from spinal to scapular)* – **6x**
- Forearm glide/stripping up over upper trapezius sliding out toward the shoulder border. – **3x**
- Double thumb glide/stripping deltoid – *(with client's arm hanging over the side of the table)*- **9x** *(Left middle and right*

aspect)

Hips

- Warm-up through the sheet. Be sure to address the outside hip muscles above the hip bone (gluteus medius and gluteus minimus)
- Deep finger kneading, starting at the sacral border from the sacrum to the hip bone. – **5x** *(slightly changing our path each time)*
- Fingertip kneading from the outer hip bone up towards the hip crest. **3x**

Tun over, Position: Face-up

Chest

- Oil On
- Warm-up
- Fist compressions to upper chest – **4x**
- Fist glide/stripping from chest to shoulder – **3x**

Arm (do both arms)

- Oil on
- Warm-up with Effleurage
- Thumb stroking to both sides of the condyle (elbow) just above the epicondyles.
- Fist glide/stripping down the front of the forearm – **3x-5x.** *You will do more work on your client's dominant arm.*
- Fist gliding/stripping down the back of the

forearm *(turn forearm)* – **3x-5x.** *Depending on your client's dominant arm, you will do more work.*

- ELD hand massage
- **Repeat on the other arm.**

Neck

- Oil on
- Warm-up
- Fingertip glide / stripping up the back of the neck with both hands – **5x**
- Fingertip kneading to the upper back of the neck just under the skull

Hockey

This is the first sport you are dealing with, where most injuries are from physical contact.

Since those are not predictable, you will base your framework for the massage on common muscles used.

*Upper body will focus on arms and chest.

The focus of the chest will be on the side of the client's shooting stance (right-handed shot = more focus on the right chest)

Your focus – Front and back of legs. Back, Shoulders, Arms, Chest, and neck.

Upper and Lower Back

- Start with a routine Swedish massage.
- Deep palmar glide/stripping up Main Erector Spinae group. – **9x** (break up back into three sections, 3x per section).
- Deep elbow glide/stripping up Main Erector Spinae group. – **9x**
- Forearm glide/stripping up over Upper Trapezius sliding out toward shoulder border. – **3x**
- Fist glide the back of the shoulder blade from the shoulder to the bottom of the shoulder blade. *(with the client's arm hanging over the side of the table)* – **5x**

Hips

- Warm-up the right hip through the sheet. This can drift upwards to include some low-back warm-ups also. Again, think about the anatomy of the hip.
  - Your focus is on the glutes and the deep supporting muscles of the hip. Be sure to address the very side of the hip, around and above the hip bone.
- Fist or elbow glide/stripping in the direction of glutes, we start at the border of the sacrum. *(Working through the sheet)* – **5x.**
- Fist or elbow glide/stripping from the sacrum to the Hip bone – **5x** *(across the hip).*
- **Repeat left side**

Back of Leg

- Oil on
- Warm-up entire leg with effleurage – **3x**
- Deep, palmer glide works the top aspect of the hamstring, both with the fiber and across – **5x**
- Supported elbow or fist glide/stripping work down the leg in 3 lines covering each line – **3x** *(9x total)*
- Beating and pounding to the whole area of the post thigh. *Make sure to address the outside edge of the thigh -* **1x**

Back of the Calf

- Deep thumb kneading over both heads of the calf. – **1x**
- Fist glide/stripping coming down both sides of the calf down to just above the Achilles tendon – **6x** *(3 per side, caution pressure at the end of stroke)*
- Deep palmar gliding at base of calf above Achilles tendon
- **Repeat on the other leg**

Turn over, Position: On Back

Chest

- Oil on
- Warm-up
- Fist compressions to upper chest – **4x**
- Fist glide/stripping from chest to shoulder – **3x**

Arms

- Oil on
- Warm-up
- Thumb stroking to both sides of the elbow, just above the epicondyles. **3x**
- Fist glide/stripping down the front of the forearm – **3x/5x** *This will depend on your client's dominant arm*
- Fist glide/stripping down the back of the forearm *(turn forearm)*– **3x/5x** *This will depend on your client's dominant arm*
- ELD hand massage

Neck

- Oil on
- Warm-up
- Fingertip glide/stripping up the back of the neck with both hands – **5x**
- Fingertip kneading to the upper back of the neck just under the skull

Racket Sport-Tennis

Tennis is both an upper and lower-body sport.

A lot of the lower body stress comes in a lateral motion.

The leg focus will be similar to hockey. However, with that lateral motion, you must focus more on the Abductors and Adductors.

Your focus – Do a Full Body Massage. Have a balanced focus between the upper and lower body.

Upper and Lower Back

- Start with a routine Swedish massage
- Deep palmar glide/stripping up Main Erector Spinae group. – **9x** *(break up back into three sections, 3x per section).*
- Deep elbow glide/stripping up Main Erector Spinae group. – **9x** *(break up back into three sections, 3x per section).*
- Forearm glide /stripping up over upper trapezius sliding out toward shoulder border. – **3x**
- Fist glide/stripping back of shoulder blade. From shoulder to the bottom of the shoulder blade *(with the client's arm hanging over the side of the table)*
- Deep thumb kneading to the back of shoulder blade and deltoids – **6x** *(3 each)*

Hips

- Warm up the hip through the sheet. This can drift upwards to include some low-back

Warm-ups also. Again, think about the anatomy of the hip.
  o Our focus is on the Glutes and the support muscles of the hip *(deep 6)*. Be sure to address the very side of the hip, around and above the hip bone
- For fist or elbow glide/stripping, we start at the border of the sacrum, moving with the direction of the Glutes (Working through the sheet). - **5x.**
- Fist or elbow glide/stripping, start at the border of the sacrum, moving with the direction of the hip bone – **5x** *(across the hip)*.

Back of the Leg

- Oil on
- Warm-up with effleurage – **3x**
- Deep palmer glide works the top aspect of the hamstring both with the fiber and across – **5x**
- Supported elbow or fist glide/stripping work down the leg in 3 lines covering each line - **3x** *(9x total)*
- Beating and pounding to the whole of the post thigh. *Make sure to address the outside edge of the thigh* - **1x**

Back of the Calf

- Deep thumb kneading over both heads of the calf. – **1x**
- Supported fist glide/stripping coming down

both sides of the calf down to just above the Achilles tendon – **6x** *(3x per side, caution pressure at the end of the stroke)*

- Deep palmar gliding at base of calf above Achilles tendon *(side to side)*
- **Repeat on the other leg**

Turn over, Position: On Back

Front of the Leg -Quads

- Oil on
- Warm-up with effleurage – **3x** upper and – **3x** lower leg.
- Deep palmar glide/stripping from hip to knee – **9x** *(3x mid and each side).*

Front of the Calf

Front and side of the calf

- Palmar glide/stripping right along the front of the shin (Tibial border) and slightly more to the outside. – 3x
- <u>Horizontal</u> fist glide/stripping at the side of the lower leg moving from knee to ankle on the outside border - 3x
- **Repeat on the other leg.**

Chest

- Oil on
- Warm-up
- Fingertip kneading compressions to the upper chest – 4x

- Fist glide/stripping from the chest to the shoulder – 3x
- Fist glide/stripping edge of pecs and front of the shoulder with fist (*with the client's arm out to side and hand raised -hello wave*) – 3x

Arms

Forearm

- Oil on
- Warm-up
- Double thumb kneading to forearm flexors.
- Fist glide/stripping along the forearm flexors from elbow to just above forearm – 5x
- *Repeat on the other arm.*

Neck

- Oil on
- Warm-up
- Fingertip glide/stripping with both hands along both sides of the neck, from base to the skull – **3x**
- Fist glide/stripping down the right side (*holding client's head in left hand*)– **3x**
- Fingertip kneading to the base of the skull.

Skiing/Snowboarding

Another majority lower body sports.

There is some nominal upper body involved for poling with skiing, and the torso is critical in turning with both skiing and snowboarding.

*The knees take the majority of abuse, so focusing around the knee will help prevent injury and enhance performance.

Your focus – Full legs. Hips and low back are essential.

With a snowboarder, identifying what stance they use (left or right leg) is worth identifying, as the rear leg works significantly harder.

Upper and Lower Back

- Start with a routine Swedish massage

Low Back

- Deep palmar glide/stripping starting at the Iliac crest, up towards the lower rib border – **4x**
- Supported fist glide/stripping just above iliac crest toward the outside of the hip – **4x**
- Beating/Pounding to the low back area and over the sheets on the glutes.

Hips

- Warm-up through sheets
- Fist or elbow glide/stripping from the top of the hip down to the upper hamstring. Moving with the direction of glutes (*Through the sheet*) – **6x**

Back of the Leg

- Oil on
- Warm-up
- Supported fist friction with and crossed fiber to the upper hamstring (origin). – **8x** (4 in each direction)
- Deep palmar glide/stripping up the hamstring – **9x** *(Separate into three sections, 3x each)*
- Fist glide/stripping along the outside aspect of the thigh – **5x** *(caution depth, the IT band can be tender)*

Back of the Calf

- Deep thumb kneading over both heads of the calf. – **1x**
- Supported fist glide/stipping down both sides of the calf down to just above the Achilles tendon – **6x** *(3 per side, caution pressure at the end of stroke)*
- Deep palmar gliding at base of calf above Achilles tendon – **4x**
- ***Repeat on the other leg***

Turn over, Position: On Back

Front of the Leg-Quads

- Oil on
- Warm-up
- Deep palmar glide/stripping starting at the hip down the thigh to the knee – **5x** (caution pressure around knee area)
- Beating and pounding, making sure to cover the entire area.
- Thumb kneading around the kneecap (*Especially at the top area of the kneecap, this feels good*). – **9x** (*3 to the left, 3 to the center, 3 to the right*)

Front of the Calf

- Supported elbow glide/stripping right along the Tibial border and slightly more to the outside. – **4x**
- ***Repeat on the other leg.***

***Finish the massage with Swedish or ELD (shoulders, arms, and face).

Soccer

Primarily a lower-body sport.

*The main injuries are in the Thighs, Feet, Knees, and Ankles (over 80% of injuries are in these areas).

With this information, it is evident that you will have 100% of our focus on the legs.

Because soccer has quite a lateral movement component, there will be more focus on the lateral calf muscle group.

Your focus – Hip, ham, calf, quads

Upper and Lower Back

- Start with a routine Swedish massage

Back of Hip

- Warm up the hip through the sheet. This can drift upwards to include some lower back Warm-ups also. Again, with the anatomy of the hip in mind, your focus is on the glutes and the supporting muscles of the hip (these muscles run from the tailbone to the outer bone of the hip).
  - Be sure to address the very side of the hip, around and above the trochanter *(thigh bone that inserts into hip bone)*
- Fist or elbow glide /stripping start at the border of the hip crest from the iliac crest down to the lower aspect of the glute *(working through the sheet)* – **5x**

- Fist or elbow glide (stripping) starts at the border of the hip crest from the iliac crest down from the sacrum to the hip bone – **5x** (across the hip).

Back of the Leg

- Oil on
- Warm-up
- Deep palmer glide work the top aspect of the hamstring, both with the fiber and across – **6x** *(3x each direction, longitudinal and across)*
- Supported elbow or fist glide/stripping work down the leg in 3 lines covering each line – **3x** (9x total)
- Beating and pounding to the whole of the post thigh. *Make sure to address all aspects of the thigh*
- Fist gliding/stripping along the outside aspect of the thigh – **3x** *(caution depth, the IT band can be tender)*

Back of the Calf

- Deep thumb kneading over both heads of the calf.
- Supported fist glide/stripping down both sides of the calf inferiorly to just above the Achilles tendon – **6x** *(3 per side, caution pressure at the end of stroke)*
- Deep palmar gliding at base of calf above Achilles tendon – **3x**
- Thumb glide/stripping along the base of the calf muscle above the Achilles

tendon - **X3**
- *Repeat on the other leg*

Turn over, Position: On Back

Front of leg-Quads

- Oil on
- Warm-up
- Deep palmar glide/stripping starting at the upper sheet border down the thigh to the knee – **5x** *(caution pressure around knee area). Change the coverage line slightly with each stroke.*
- Beating and pounding to the front of the thigh, covering the entire area.
- Thumb kneading around the kneecap *(especially at the top area of the kneecap, this feels good).* – **9x** *(3x to left, 3x to center, 3x to the right)*

Front and Side of the Calf

- Supported elbow glide/stripping to both, right along the Tibial border and slightly more laterally – **5x**
- Horizontal fist glide/stripping at the side of the lower leg moving from the knee to the ankle on the outside border – **3x**
- Double thumb kneading up the front and side of the shin
- *Repeat on the other leg*

***Finish the massage with Swedish or ELD (shoulders, arms, and face).

Swimming

Swimming is very easy on the body as far as joint impact is concerned.

Due to the various movements, this framework will be very similar to a full-body massage.

*The shoulder is the most common injury, but it is mostly isolated to competitive swimmers logging a lot of distance.

Basic Framework – even between the upper and lower body. Due to the variety of swim strokes people can choose from, we must consider the entire leg while working on the legs.

The main focus of the leg treatment will be the Quads, Hams, and Hips.

We will touch on the whole back, but the focus will be on the upper back and neck junction and the shoulder. This is due to most body positions involving a head-up position and the extensive range of motion concerned with the shoulder.

Upper and Lower Back

- Start with a routine Swedish massage.
- Deep palmar glide/stripping starting at *Mid-back up to the neck* – **6x** (*divide in half, 3x each*)
- Thumb glide/stripping from the spinal border of the scapula towards and/or away from the spine – **3x**
- Thumb glide/stripping from the spinal

border of the scapula towards the neck (*45-degree angle up*) – **3x**

- Elbow glide/stripping up over the trapezius sweeping out towards shoulder – **5x**
- Fist glide/stripping back of the shoulder blade from the shoulder to the bottom of the shoulder blade (*with the client's arm hanging over the side of the table*) – **5x**
- Double thumb glide/stripping the deltoid (*with client arm hanging over the side of the table*) – **9x** (*Left middle and right aspect*)

Hips

- Warm up through the sheet.
- Fist or elbow glide/stripping start at the border of the sacrum, moving with the direction of the glutes (*Working through the sheet*) - **5x**
- Fist or elbow glide/stripping from the sacrum to the Hip bone – **5x** (*across the hip*).

Back of the Leg

- Oil on
- Warm-up with effleurage – **3x**
- Deep palmer glide work the top aspect of the hamstring both with the fiber and across – **6x** (*3x each direction; longitudinal and across*)
- Supported elbow or fist glide/stripping, work down the leg in 3 lines covering each line – **3x** (*9x total*)

- Beating and pounding to the whole of the post thigh. *Make sure to address the outside edge of the thigh.*

Back of the Calf

- Deep thumb kneading over both heads of the calf. **– 1x**
- Supported fist glide/stripping down both sides of the calf down to just above the Achilles tendon **– 6x** *(3x per side, caution pressure at the end of stroke)*
- Deep palmar gliding at the base of calf above Achilles tendon **– 4x**
- **Repeat on the other leg**

Turn over, Position: On Back

Front of the leg-Quads

- Oil on
- Warm-up
- Deep palmar glide/stripping starting at the hip down the thigh to the knee **– 5x** (caution pressure around knee area)
- Beating and pounding the front quads making sure to cover the entire area.
- Thumb kneading around the kneecap (especially at the top area of the kneecap, this feels good). **– 9x** *(3x to left, 3x to center, 3x to the right)*

Front of calf

- Supported elbow glide/stripping right along

the Tibia border and slightly more to the outside. - **X4**

- ***Repeat on the other leg.***

Neck

- Oil on
- Warm-up
- Fingertip glide/stripping up the back of the neck with both hands – **5x**
- Fingertip kneading to the upper back of the neck just under the skull.

Abdomen/Stomach Massage

Procedure:

- Oil on
- General Effleurage (warms up the stomach to get ready for the rest of the moves)
- The following three movements of the stomach are moving the digestive system, which runs from the person's right side hip to leg, across from right to left, and down hip to leg left side.
  - The large intestine (large colon) is like an upside-down u shape.
  - If you go slow enough, you can sometimes feel blocked food, which can move. Again, this is an excellent part of the massage for healing purposes.
- The next step is circles using both hands. (still working on the large intestine)
- Dein Tan is an Energy move (waiting for the client to take a breath)
- Side pulls and fan (is now working on getting the lymph from the back of the body to the center of the stomach)
- General Effleurage (just relaxing the stomach after working it)

Back, Neck, and Shoulder Massage

Procedure:

The client is in the prone position *(facing down)*

- Put a small amount of Shea butter or cream on your hand
- Rub together to liquefy
- Apply to the appropriate area on the client (if your hands are cold, touch with forearm first)
- Repeat as needed

Upper and Lower Back

a. **Choose one side first**
Start with a routine Swedish massage to warm the body up.

- Effleurage
- Feather strokes
- Open C's
- 3 – 5 minutes Warm-up of the whole area.

Hand

a. Start with fast hand glides (fanning) **3x**
b. Slow the hand glides down and put more pressure **3x**
c. Your hand at 45 ° (go slow) double hand

glide with pressure to as close to a grade 5-9
3x

Thumb

d. Side to side **3x**
e. Karate chop motion (wax on, wax off) **3x**

f. Push up **3x**

Knuckles

g. Flat glide *-can reinforce* **3x** (knuckles down)
h. Circles **3x**
i. Ulna side glide **3x**
j. Friction glide **3x**

Forearm

k. Flat glide (whole arm -finger to elbow) **3x each row (rows of three)**

Elbow (Maybe too deep for some clients)

l. Reinforced elbow glide **3x each row (rows of three)**

Edge of Spine *(intent is on the edge of spine)*

Hand

m. Start with fast hand glides (fanning) **3x**
n. Slow the hand glides down and put more pressure **3x**
o. Your hand is at 45 ° (go slow). Double hand glide with pressure to as close to a grade 5-9 **3x**

Thumb

    p. Side to side   **3x**

    q. Karate chop motion (wax on, wax off) **3x**

    r. Push up **3x**

Knuckles

    s. Flat glide -*can reinforce* **3x** (knuckles down)

    t. Circles **3x**

    u. Ulna side glide **3x**

    v. Friction glide **3x**

Forearm

    w. Flat glide (whole arm -finger to elbow) **3x each row (rows of three)**

Elbow (Maybe too deep for some clients)

    x. Reinforced elbow glide **3x each row (rows of three)**

Switch to the other side - Repeat

Start with a routine Swedish massage to warm the body up.

- Effleurage
- Feather strokes
- Open C`s
- 3 – 5 minutes Warm-up of the whole area.

Hand

   a. Start with fast hand glides (fanning) **3x**
   b. Slow the hand glides down and put more pressure **3x**
   c. Hand at 45 ° (go slow) double hand glide with pressure to as close to a grade 5-9 **3x**

Thumb

   d. Side to side   **3x**
   e. Karate chop motion (wax on, wax off) **3x**

   f. Push up **3x**

Knuckles

   g. Flat glide *-can reinforce* **3x** (knuckles down)
   h. Circles **3x**
   i. Ulna side glide **3x**
   j. Friction glide **3x**

Forearm

   k. Flat glide (whole arm -finger to elbow) **3x each row (rows of three)**

Elbow (Maybe too deep for some clients)

   l. Reinforced elbow glide **3x each row (rows of three)**

Edge of Spine *(intent is on the edge of spine)*

Hand

    m. Start with fast hand glides (fanning) **3x**

    n. Slow the hand glides down and put more pressure **3x**

    o. Hand at 45 ° (go slow) double hand glide with pressure to as close to a grade 5-9 **3x**

Thumb

    p. Side to side **3x**

    q. Karate chop motion (wax on, wax off) **3x**

    r. Push up **3x**

Knuckles

    s. Flat glide *-can reinforce* **3x** (knuckles down)

    t. Circles **3x**

    u. Ulna side glide **3x**

    v. Friction glide **3x**

Forearm

    w. Flat glide (whole arm -finger to elbow) **3x each row (rows of three)**

Elbow (Maybe too deep for some clients)

    x. Reinforced elbow glide **3x each row (rows of three)**

Shift to the opposite side of the neck (from the side of the back you were just on)

Warm the neck up.

- 3 – 5 minutes Warm-up of the whole area.

Hand

a. Start with lighter fast hand glides (shoulder to ear) **3x**
b. Slow the hand glides down and put more pressure (shoulder to the neck)**3x**

Thumb

c. Side to side **3x**
d. Karate chop motion (wax on, wax off) **3x**

e. Push up **3x**

Knuckles

f. Flat glide -*can reinforce* **3x** (knuckles down)
g. Circles **3x**

Forearm

h. Glide **3x**

Shift to the opposite side of the neck

Warm the neck up.

- 3 – 5 minutes Warm-up of the whole area.

Hand

i. Start with lighter fast hand glides (shoulder to the ear) **3x**
j. Slow the hand glides down and put more pressure (shoulder to the neck)**3x**

Hand

a. Start with quick hand glides (fanning) **3x**
b. Slow the hand glides down and put more pressure **3x**
c. Hand at 45 ° (go slow) double hand glide with pressure to as close to a grade 5-9 **3x**

Thumb

d. Side to side **3x**
e. Karate chop motion (wax on, wax off) **3x**

f. Push up **3x**

Knuckles

g. Flat glide -*can reinforce* **3x** (knuckles down)
h. Circles **3x**

Forearm

i. Glide **3x**

Breast Massage

Function

The function of the breasts is lactation.

Structure

The breasts are located over the pectoral muscles and are attached to them by connective tissue. Each breast comprises 15 - 20 lobes of glandular tissue that can produce milk. In addition, each lobe opens into a duct, which empties through the nipple. Therefore, each breast has approximately 15 to 20 openings.

The breast has adipose tissue surrounding the lobes. The amount of tissue determines the size of the breasts. However, size plays no role in milk production.

The nipple consists of smooth muscle that can contract. In addition, several rudimentary milk glands are located in the areola surrounding the nipple.

High concentrations of estrogen and progesterone stimulate the glands and ducts during pregnancy. This results in increased breast size. After birth, the breasts release colostrum, which contains protein and lactose with little fat. In addition, the suckling stimulation causes the endocrine system's pituitary to release **oxytocin and prolactin.** Oxytocin causes the breasts to release milk.

Lymph Node Areas Adjacent to the Breast Area

Pectoralis major muscle

Axillary lymph nodes: level I

Axillary lymph nodes: level II

Axillary lymph nodes: level III

Supraclavicular lymph nodes

Internal mammary lymph nodes

Check to see if the client wears an under-wire bra. The wire can be an issue because the metal can act as a magnet and attract energy to the breasts, creating fascia adhesion. Also, a bra or sports bra is tight, and the lymph never moves correctly while the bra is worn. Even worse, if the person sleeps in their bra or a tight shirt.

Remind the person to take off their bra when they get home and are going nowhere. This allows the breast to move while walking around; once they go to bed, the lymph will not have a chance to move.

The breast is not connected to the rib cage; it is floating on the fascia.

Mastectomy
When a breast has been removed, the client may have double removed both breasts.

Breast Implants
If the client has silicon or similar implants, <u>do</u> <u>not</u> massage.

Breast reduction is not usually a lot of scarring and can heal very well. Proceed to the procedure section.

Very important to massage the tissue: from the wrist, inside of the elbow, underarm, and breast area.

Once the surgery is eight weeks old, and the client has permission from their Doctor for massage, you can proceed.

Some clients have some stomach muscle removed and moved up into the breast area, with a nipple made from their skin tissue being tucked around and tattooed to create an areola.

Once you have Doctor's permission to massage, proceed similarly to the lymphatic massage procedure.

Chemotherapy affects all cells in the body.
Radiotherapy creates scarring for the rest of the person's life.

Types of Breast Surgery
1) **A biopsy** is a kind of surgery that will create scarring. Some women have as many as 18 different entries. It can be worse than the surgery – physiological trauma
2) **Lump removed and nodes** – will minimize arm movement.
3) **Partial Mastectomy** – only part of the breast tissue is removed and usually replaced with tissue from the thigh (Now you have two areas that need fascia work).
4) **Total Mastectomy** – the entire breast is removed down to the ribs, including all lymph nodes (women do this for fear of cancer returning). Then, the surgeon has to create skin flaps that are widened for the removal being done underneath. Usually, Teres minor and major are also cut into and some removed.

5) **Liposuction** may be done on the opposite breast to create similar sizing. It has been proven that the fat will come back anyways.
6) Or increase an area with fat from another body part, usually the leg.

Scarring usually creates issues with the fascia connecting to the bone and muscle, and the skin will not move/flex properly. Fatty tissue is generally removed. The layers adhere to each other.

Some scars are so bad that only surgery can release the tissue.

Lymph drainage is an excellent technique for people with Fibroids, Cancer, and Lymphatic Drainage issues.

Different size breasts will be done all the same.

LYMPHATIC BREAST MASSAGE PROCEDURE

The pressure of movement is very light and slow.

Cover one breast while working on the other.

Step 1: 3 sets

Position your hand on the side to be worked on (this position does not touch the nipple). The hand is sidewise with the pointer finger and thumb spread out and touching the skin.

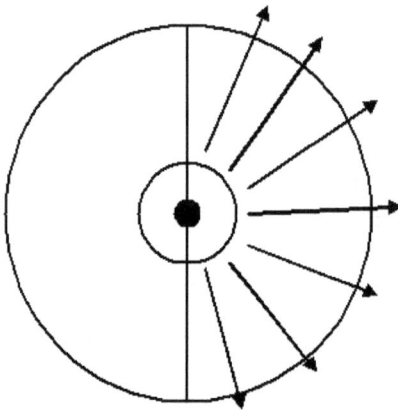

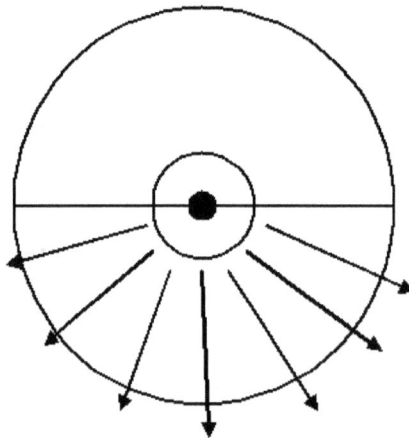

Hold the working hand with two or three fingers.

Move from the center of the breast, approximately six moves.

Step 2: 3 sets

Position your hand on the side to be worked on (this position does not touch the nipple). The hand is sidewise with the pointer finger and thumb spread out and touching the skin.

Hold the working hand with two or three fingers.

Move from the center of the breast, approximately six moves.

Step 3: 3 sets

Position your holding hand on the side to be worked on (this position does not touch the nipple). The hand is sidewise with the pointer finger and thumb spread out and touching the skin.

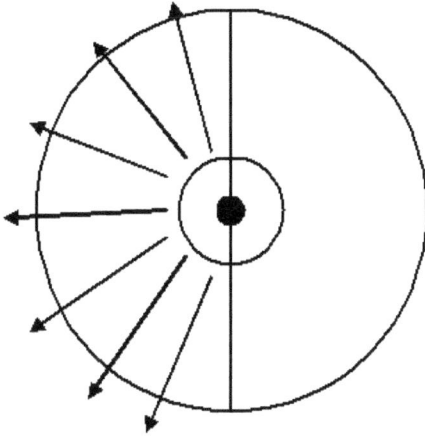

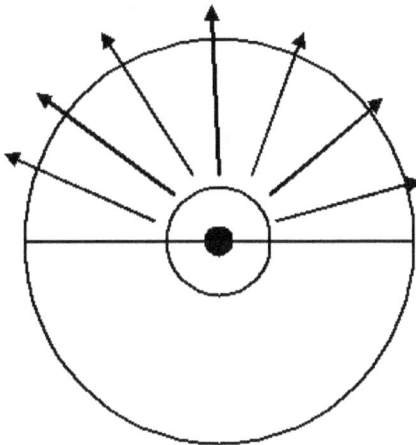

Hold the working hand with two or three fingers.

Move from the center of the breast, approximately six moves.

Step 4: 3 sets

Position your holding hand on the side to be worked on (this position does not touch the nipple). The hand is sidewise with the pointer finger and thumb spread out and touching the skin.

Hold the working hand with two or three fingers.

Move from the center of the breast, approximately six moves.

Step 5: 3 sets

Massage with both hands around the breast area to the lines from the upper center. 3-5x

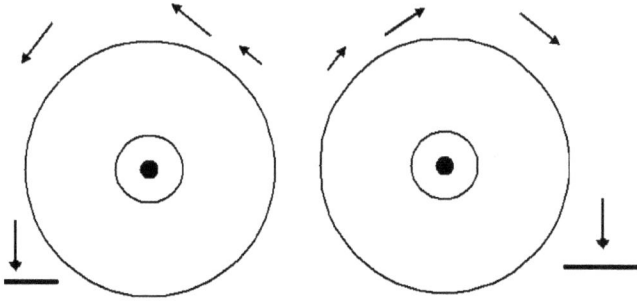

Step 6: 3 sets

Massage with both hands around the breast area to the lines from the center medial. 3-5x

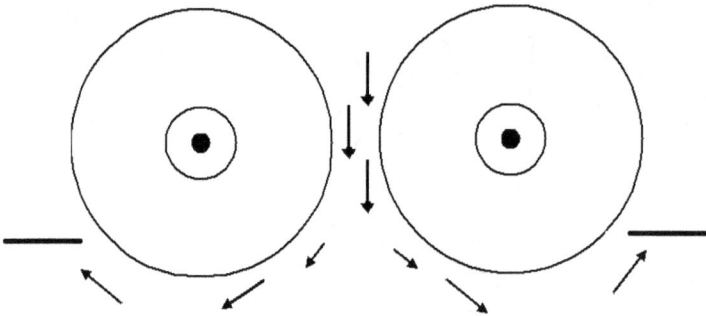

If you have taken the Aromatherapy course, you can massage with an essential oil blend.

Carrier Oil: Grapeseed, jojoba, and olive can be used.

Castor oil is an excellent carrier/massage oil but can stain clothing, ask the client to wear something. They do not care if oil gets on it.

Castor oil helps to dissolve fibroids and change cell memory.

Extra step:

After the massage, saturate white cotton cloth (big enough to cover both breasts) and lay on the breast area. Saran wrap around the client's body -breast area covered top and bottom (not too tightly), so no oil can seep out and have them lay there for 30 minutes.

Remove the wrap and cloth and have clients lightly wipe away excess oil.

Have the client do this at home but to sleep wrapped up, 3-4 nights in a row. Add more oil to the white cotton cloth each night and re-wrap it with the new wrap.

Tell clients that bedding might get stained, so do not use good sheets.

Mastectomy massage procedure:

- **Great to do a full body massage; do arms, shoulders, and face and then come back to breasts**
- Check movement and where the fascia is.
- Check the neck as well up to cheeks
- Massage the scarring and fascia only to the client's pain tolerance, maybe only a 3.

Chair Massage

Why Chair Massage?

There are many advantages to practicing Chair Massage.

It is convenient for people in working clothes and a business environment. In addition, a sitting position makes it easy and accessible, especially for people who are conventional, elderly, pregnant, overweight or have no prior massage experience.

Practitioners worldwide can set up a business in an airport, train station, bus station, mall, outdoor booth (park or beach), trade show, farmers fair, and mobile, in an office, hospital, care unit, or school. *You will need a business license, permit, and liability insurance.*

Two minutes to thirty minutes is the average time frame of a session.

You can use any Swedish Massage Technique, but the following procedures use Shiatsu's acupressure Techniques.

2 Minute Massage

(Great for trade show free demos)

Have the client sit comfortably.

> Knead the Shoulders: 3-5 times (x)
>> Place both hands on the tops of the shoulders near the base of the neck and firmly massage them in slow motion.
>>
>> *Ask how the depth of pressure feels to get the client's feedback.*

> Thumb down the upper back: 1-3x
>> Keep your fingers on the tops of the shoulders, and use your thumbs to press between the spine and shoulder blades firmly. The practitioner should have one leg back and one leg forward, rocking their weight back and forth, leaning into the upper back with the thumbs.

> Thumb and Bent Finger Squeeze: 1-3x
>> Brace the front of the chest or shoulder with one hand and continue a light pinch down the spine.

> Energy Brushing: 3x
>> Gently run your fingertips over the crown of the head and down your client's back.

Repeat any of the moves if the timing is too fast.

5 Minute Massage

Have the client sit comfortably.

Knead the Shoulders: 3-5 (x)
> Place both hands on the tops of the shoulders near the base of the neck and firmly massage them in slow motion.

Energy Brushing: 1-3x
> Gently run your fingertips over the crown of the head and down your client's back.

Apply firm pressure with the flat of your fists down and inward on the top of the shoulders.

Thumb down the whole back: 1-3x
> Move down to the sacrum using your thumbs to firmly press along the outside of the spine. The practitioner should have one leg back and one leg forward, rocking their weight back and forth, leaning into the upper back with the thumbs.

Neck Press: 8-10x
> Gently press the back of the head downward. Next, interlock your fingers or place one hand over the other, using the heel of your hands to press out the tension on each side of the neck.

"Gates of Consciousness" (Gall Bladder Meridian 20 –GB20): 3x
> Position your fingertips on one side, your thumb on the other, into the hollows behind the ears. Slowly till the head,

applying pressure upward as you lightly
squeeze your thumbs and fingers together.

Energy Brushing: 3x
Gently run your fingertips over the crown
of the head and down your client's back.

As you slowly take your hands off the body, encourage
the client to keep their eyes closed and relax for a few
more moments.

10 Minute Massage

Have the client sit comfortably.

Knead the Shoulders: 8-10x
> Place both hands on the tops of the
> shoulders near the base of the neck and
> firmly massage them in slow motion.

Energy Brushing: 1-3x
> Gently run your fingertips over the crown
> of the head and down your client's back.

Thumb down the whole back: 1-3x
> Move down to the sacrum using your
> thumbs to firmly press along the outside of
> the spine. The practitioner should have one
> leg back and one leg forward, rocking their
> weight back and forth, leaning into the
> upper back with the thumbs.

Thumb and Bent Finger Squeeze: 3x
> Brace the front of the chest or shoulder with
> one hand and continue a light pinch down the
> spine.

Slowly Lean Your Fists into the Top of the
Shoulders: 8-10x
> Stand close so that your front is touching
> the back of your client. It often helps to
> stand up on your toes to get the leverage to
> gradually apply firm pressure to the
> shoulder (trapezius) muscles. You can also
> do this from the front of the client.

Neck Press: 8-10x
>
> Gently press the back of the head downward.
> Next, interlock your fingers or place one
> hand over the other, using the heel of your
> hands to press out the tension on each side of
> the neck.

Thumb down the upper back: 4-6x
>
> Keep your fingers on the tops of the
> shoulders and use your thumbs to press
> firmly between the spine and shoulder
> blades. The practitioner should have one leg
> back and one leg forward, rocking their
> weight back and forth, leaning into the
> upper back with the thumbs.

"Gates of Consciousness" (Gall Bladder Meridian
20): 3-5x
>
> Position your fingertips on one side, your
> thumb on the other, into the hollows
> behind the ears. Slowly till the head back,
> applying pressure upward as you squeeze
> your thumbs and fingers together.

Energy Brushing: 3x
>
> Gently run your fingertips over the crown
> of the head and down your client's back.

As you slowly take your hands off the body, encourage
the client to keep their eyes closed and relax for a few
more moments.

15 Minute Massage

Have the client sit comfortably.

Knead the Shoulders: 3-5 times (x)
> Place both hands on the tops of the
> shoulders near the base of the neck and
> firmly massage them in slow motion.

Energy Brushing: 1-3x
> Gently run your fingertips over the crown
> of the head and down your client's back.

Hack 3-5x each side
> Lightly karate chops the trapezius
> muscles (shoulders).

Energy Brushing: 1-3x
> Gently run your fingertips over the crown
> of the head and down your client's back.

Shoulders: 3-4x
> Apply firm pressure with the flat of your
> fists down and inward on the top of the
> shoulders.

Thumb down the whole back: 1-3x
> Move down to the sacrum using your
> thumbs to firmly press along the outside of
> the spine. The practitioner should have one
> leg back and one leg forward, rocking their
> weight back and forth, leaning into the
> upper back with the thumbs.

Sacrum Squeeze. 3x
> Interlock your fingers and squeeze the
> lower back (lumbar and sacrum).

Raising the Shoulders. 3x
> Place one hand on each shoulder, lightly lift
> and release.

Energy sweeps the Shoulder 1-3x
> From shoulders down to the upper arms.

Stand or kneel in front and continue.

"Elegant Mansion" (Kidney meridian 27) 3x
> Lightly press the thumb and pointer finger
> > into the Kidney meridian 27.
> Just under the collarbone, either side of the
> sternum. Should feel two indents

"Letting Go "Lung l meridian 3x
> It is located on the outer side of the chest,
> three finger-widths below the collarbone,
> closer to the armpits.

Arms 3x
> Squeeze down the entire arm, both sides.

Hands and fingers 1-3x
> Massage the hand by lightly rubbing your
> palm and lightly massaging and pulling the
> fingers.

Squeeze upper Legs 3x
>Even squeeze over the tops of thighs.

Energy Brushing 3-5x
>Gently run your fingertips over the crown
>of the head and down your client's back.

Vibrate down the spine 3x

>Hold the client with one hand on their
>shoulder while the other is lightly shaking
>back and forth down the spine.

As you slowly take your hands off the body, encourage
the client to keep their eyes closed and relax for a few
more moments.

Facial Massage

I usually do not put more cream or oil on my hands for the face. Instead, I use whatever is left on my hands from the massage or nothing.

Spa Facial

- Massage shoulders
- Lightly tap, tap, tap along jawline – right to left, and back 3x
- Tap, tap, stroke on right cheek - walk over chin – tap, tap, stroke on left cheek 3x
- Effleurage sweeping strokes to the hairline, across the forehead 3x
- Forehead circles, one side to the other, three lines 3x
- Forehead - criss-cross x - across 3x
- Using middle finger, circles around eyes 3x
- Light tap around eyes 3x
- Starting from above the nose at the brow, light circles under the eyes, glide back up 3x
- Using your hand, glide along the jawline, each direction 3x
- Light tap around cheeks 3x (I use three fingers on each side)
- Circles, edge of the face to under the nose, glide back, edge of the face to the edges of the mouth,

glide back, from the edge of the face to the chin, glide back 3x

- Finger sweep across the upper lip (switch hands), finger sweep across the chin (switch hands) 3x
- Start at the chin, one hand at each side, glide around the chin, glide around the mouth to under the nose and back 3x
- Sweep under the chin at the neckline 3x
- Effleurage down the neck, one side, and then the other 3x
- Glide up the side of the face and effleurage sweeping strokes to the hairline, across the forehead 3x

Hand Massage

Apply oil or cream to your hands.

- Taking one of their hand, slowly pancake over – one hand on either side (turn over to reveal palm)

ALWAYS Protect their wrist with your fingers

- Holding one of your hands under their wrist, fan wrist with your other hand's thumb 3x
- Fan the palm alternating thumb sweeps (your fingers are under them) 3x
- Using your thumbs, small circle movements over their palm 3x
- Hook your pinkie fingers down through their thumb and pinkie, light stretch, light stroking motion using your thumbs 3x
- Using your finger and thumb, massage each finger 1x

Pancake – one hand on either side (turn over to reveal the dorsal side/back of the hand)

- Your fingers holding their weight, use your thumbs to create circles (finger base to wrist) 3x
- Using your finger and thumb, massage each finger 1x
- Using your thumbs, fan the dorsal side of their hand 3x

Place their hand on the abdomen or beside them.

Repeat, on the other hand.

Hot Stone Massage

Heat is excellent for relaxing chronic, tight, and sore muscles
but <u>Contra-indicated</u> for (cannot do on people):

***Very important! **Check** contra-indications!!!!
If not, you cannot massage them with heated stones.

Contra-indicated for:

- Inflammation
- Pregnancy
- Diabetes
- Neuropathy
- Nerve surgery
- Some prescription medication
- Obese/overweight
- Heart disease or issues
- Varicose veins
- All autoimmune dysfunctions (chronic fatigue)
- Thin skin (elderly or very young)

The best question to ask is,
"Can you fully submerge in a hot tub for 20 minutes?"
If yes, then you can use hot stones.

Equipment Needed

- Crockpot (heater)
- Water temperature 120°F / 49°C – to a max of 135°F / 57°C
- Basalt stone (lave rocks)
  - 8 toe stones (diameter approx. ¾" - 1" / 1.9cm - 2.5 cm)
  - 14-18 small stones (diameter approx. 1" - 2" / 2.5 cm- 5 cm)
  - 18-20 medium stones (diameter approx. 2" - 3" / 5 cm – 7.5cm)
  - 6-8 large stones (diameter approx. 3" - 4" / 7.5cm – 10 cm)
- Massage oil – (Holly glides great when heated)
- Plastic serrated (holes) spoon
- Sheet set (towel like Swedish Massage)
- Four hand towels – one for the basket, one for the belly/ breast, one for back stones, and one for your hands to dry and carry stones.
- Basket or bowl (for used stones)

Set-up: table- fitted sheet and cover, might also need blanket and pillows
- jewelry needs to be removed (metal can burn when heated)

Time: One-hour booking- (hands-on approx. 50 min and 5 min on / 5 min off)

Procedure: If someone has an inflamed or swollen area and does not need a Doctor, you can use cold stones to help reduce the swelling.

Cold stones are kept in the freezer and can be used on the area with a Kleenex or sheet, laid down first, or used in the massage with the oil. You can combine the massage with one cold stone and one hot stone or both cold. Use very sparingly and for specific areas. Many people hate the feeling of cold on them. Always! Check with the client before using it.

Hot stones are heated in the crockpot. I layer the lava stones in a specific size so I do not make so much noise during the massage. I fill the crockpot almost full of hot water and then add the rest with boiled water from a kettle. For the rest of the session, put the lid on, and turn to the lowest temperature on the crockpot.

Remember, **if you <u>cannot</u> touch the stones, your client cannot have them on their body! So** I bring a rock or two out, DRY them off and get to the massage table.
<u>If</u> the stone is too hot, I warm my hands and place the rocks away from the client's skin on the table. Then, I start to massage the area with my warm hands, and when the stone is ready, I bring it into the massage with smooth gliding strokes in a general effleurage technique.

The stones will cool quickly; you can turn them in your hands to help cool them faster or use the other side. The person's body will take and absorb the heat.
The pressure will be very light. You are not to apply extra pressure to let the heat of the stone do the work.
Stay off of any bony area. Massage the muscles only.

Hot Stone Session:

Back
>· Place 1 small stone in the center of the towel and give it to the client to place under themselves at the belly button area.
>· Place 1 medium to large stone on the lower back on top of the sheet
>· Lower the sheet covering them to reveal their back
>· Oil on
>· 2 medium stones (*can get 2 more if they cool too quickly*)
>· Start the massage with effleurage strokes, and if stones are ready to use right away
>· You can move in any direction and also in circles
>· Time is about 5-10 min max

Arms- back of
>· Oil on
>· Can do with 1 small stone
>· Time is one minute for each arm
>· Leave the stone in hand
>· Repeat on the other arm

Back Leg
>· Reveal one leg
>· Oil on
>· 2 medium stones
>· Time is max 4-5 minutes
>· Repeat on the other leg

Remove all stones and turn the client over.

Have the client sit up and place the six large stones on the table, cover the stones with a towel, and help the client lie down. *Ensure there is lots of room for their spine (the spine should never touch the stones).*

On the front of the client's chest chakra area
- Place small to medium stones on the heart, solar plexus, sacral chakra area
- New stone in each hand

Front Legs
- Reveal leg
- Oil on
- 2 medium stones massage leg
- Time is max 4-5 minutes
- Repeat on the other leg
- Place toe stones in on both feet (make sure they are not too hot)

Stomach
- Remove chakra stones
- Reveal stomach
- Oil on
- 2 small/medium stones
- Time is max 4-5 minutes
- Can leave more stones on chakra

Shoulders
- Reveal area
- Oil on
- 2 small/medium stones
- Massage area
- Time is max 4-5 minutes
- Can leave stones under soft-spot behind shoulders

Arms
- Remove the stone from the hand
- Reveal arm
- Oil on
- 2 small/medium stones massage arm and hand
- Time is maxed at 5 minutes
- Repeat on the other arm
- Can leave a stone in the hand

Face
> · 1 small stone
> · Rub stone in your hands for oil (no extra oil needed)
> · Massage face slowly

Remove all stones, and ask if the client needs help turning over or getting off the table.

Clean up:
> · Take all stones and put them in the sink (make sure toe stones cannot go down the drain).
> · Wash with soap and water
> · Rinse
> · Put on a towel / dry
> · Spray both sides with rubbing alcohol

Not necessary to put oil back on the stones. Oil can go rancid (especially if heated), so be careful how long the stones are left between sessions if using oil between uses.

Lymph Drainage Massage

Why do a Lymph Drainage Massage?

The lymphatic system has no heart to pump the fluid by itself. It needs movement. Walking, jumping, deep breathing, and manual massage help to move lymph.

Lymph

- destroying waste,
- debris,
- dead blood cells,
- pathogens,
- toxins,
- and cancer cells,
- absorbs fats and fat-soluble vitamins from the digestive system,
- removes excess fluid and waste products from the interstitial spaces between the cells,
- and works with your immune system.

The lymphatic system is a one-way system –

Carrying the body's waste toward the heart! Gravity is the lymph system's enemy! The lymph needs to move from the head down (not a problem), but it must move from your toes and fingertips up to the ducts just below your shoulders.

The lymphatic system has two main ducts: the left and right.

Location – see
Bullseye

The fascinating part is
that the smaller duct,
the **right lymphatic
duct,** receives lymph
from ONLY:

- Split the head in
  half - the right
  side of the head
  and neck only,
- The right arm
  only,
- The right side
  of the chest and back – partial only,
- It empties into the junction of the right internal
  jugular and the right subclavian vein.

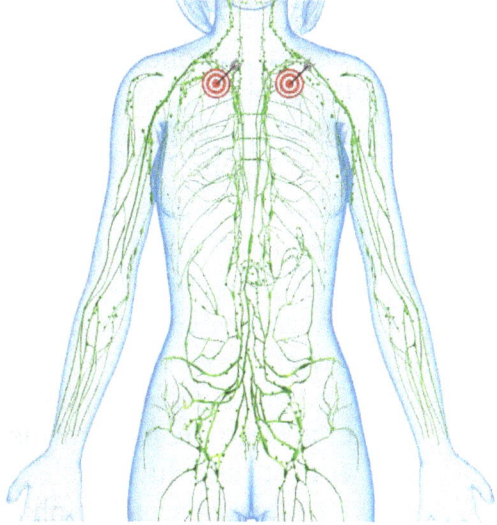

The left lymphatic or thoracic duct receives lymph from
EVERYWHERE else:

- the left side of the head and neck,
- the left side of the thorax,
- the left arm,
- AND HIPS, BUTTOCKS, and BOTH LEGS
- It empties into the junction of the left internal
  jugular and left subclavian veins.

Imagine lymph as garbage cans that you have in your
house. You have smaller garbage cans in your bedroom,
office, and bathroom. Imagine the lymph nodes inside

your elbows, underarms, breasts, behind your knees, groin, and neck as these little garbage cans.

- The knees collect the garbage from your feet to your knees.
- The groin collects the garbage from your knees to the groin.
- The groin collects the lymph and sends it to the cisterna chyli and then to the left lymphatic duct ONLY.
- The neck collects the lymph from your head and face, then goes to the appropriate duct.
- The elbow collects the garbage from your hands to the elbows.
- The underarms collect the garbage from your elbows to the underarms, then goes to the appropriate duct.
- Each breast area lymph then goes to the appropriate duct.
- Both ducts drain 90 % of fluid back to the circulatory system and 10% of fluid to the digestive system to be eliminated.

Enfleurage - stroking movements. This is usually the main movement of the body. Use your palms and fingers. It can include:
- **Gliding**
- **Sweeping**
- **Fanning**

***To move lymph, the secret is the pressure used. THE WEIGHT OF A NICKEL – <u>very</u> light pressure, soft as a feather!!!

Procedure:
- Pump 3x with an open palm, both the left and right duct.

From here, you can decide on what part of the body you want to start with.

ALWAYS drain towards the heart!!!

- Back of body to the front (follow ribs)
- Front of the legs to the back of the leg
- Back of the ankles to behind the knees
- Behind the knees to the inside of the groin
- Groin to below the ribs to the sternum
- Fingers to the elbows
- Elbows to the underarm
- Underarm to the breast
- Breast to below the ribs to the sternum
- Face – the center of the face to below the ear
- Below the ear down the neck
- Décolletage around the outside of the breast to below the ribs to the sternum

Motion of movement
- Pump 3x with an open palm, both the left and right duct.
- Each movement is snail-slow sweeping strokes in a line from point A to B
- Example: thumb fan (one thumb at a time – barely touching the person!) from ankle to knee in a straight line. It is going to take many lines to do the full calf.
- Repeat 3x, and move very SLOWLY!!!
- Then move up to do the back of the leg – same many lines from knee to groin.
- Arms
- Breasts (see breast massage)
- Face

- End - Pump 3x with an open palm, both the left and right duct.

Pregnancy Massage

Many pregnant women have many aches and pains due to their bodies changing weight so fast.

Sore backs are the most common complaint from the body's new weight, and skin stretching is next.

Massage is a beautiful way to help the client release some pain from both issues.

Most pregnant women love massage for its benefit on the digestive, circulation, and lymphatic systems. And many say they sleep well for a couple of days after a massage.

Perfect for the partner to learn how to help alleviate the pain before and during labor pains or Broxton Hicks contractions.

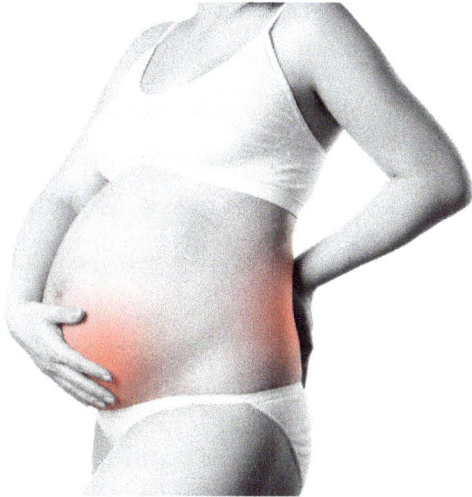

Equipment:

Most practitioners use a regular massage table with many pillows. However, you can purchase specially made massage tables with a hollow for the big tummy and breast area.
You can also use a chair massage position.

Anatomy- Fetus Development
Quick Reference
First trimester
Zero – Two months in the womb is considered a Fetus/embryo.
23 days heartbeat
Two months the baby is the size of a kidney bean and has slightly webbed fingers
11 weeks baby can suck its thumb
Three months 7-8 centimeters (3 inches) big

Second trimester
Four months 13 centimeters (5 ½ inches) big
Most women start to show up at this stage. Their tummies grow fast after this.
Five months eyebrows and lashes are there now and 27 centimeters (10.5 inches)
a mother can feel the baby kick
Six months Baby weighs 660 grams or 1.5 pounds

Third trimester
Seven months 40 centimeters (15 inches) big, can open eyes
Eight months Baby weighs 2.2 kg or 4.7 pounds. Lungs are developed.
Nine Months 50 centimeters (20.5 inches) big, Baby weighs 3.4 kg or 7.5 pounds.

BASIC PREGNANCY MASSAGE PROCEDURE:

Position the client in <u>their</u> most comfortable position. You will do similar movements to the European Lymph Drainage Massage and Swedish (free flow) Techniques.

Use only easy moves that cannot cause any pain to the client!!!

The client may be lying on her side with a pillow or two between her legs (she will tell you what is best)

Upper and Lower back
- Change towel
- Effleurage   3-5x
- Feathers   3x each side
- Rainbows   1 set
- Drain 2x
- Repeat Rainbows   1 set
- Drain 2x
- Open 'C' all over back
- Shoulders drain with arm 3x each arm
- Finish with Effleurage moves to drain Lymph

Back Legs: Lower and Upper
First leg
- Change towel
- Effleurage from foot to thigh   3x
- Free flow moves - e.g., Open 'c' or kneading
- Lower calf drain
- Knee
- Finish with Effleurage moves to drain Lymph

Second leg
- Effleurage from foot to thigh   3x
- Free flow moves - e.g., Open 'c' or kneading
- Lower calf drain
- Knee
- Finish with Effleurage moves to drain Lymph
- Change towel

Turn clients over may need many pillows under their legs to take the pressure off their lower back.

Front Legs: Lower and Upper

First leg
- Change towel
- Effleurage from foot to thigh 3x
- Inner leg from thigh to foot
- Free flow moves - e.g., Open 'c' or kneading
- Inner inguinal drain
- Knee
- Finish with Effleurage moves to drain Lymph

Second leg
- Effleurage from foot to thigh 3x
- Inner leg from thigh to foot
- Free flow moves - e.g., Open 'c' or kneading
- Inner inguinal drain
- Knee
- Finish with Effleurage moves to drain Lymph
- Change towel

Tummy (great feeling for you and the client- Baby lots of time follows you with a foot or hand)
- Change towel
- Follow the procedure for the ELD massage
  - Oil on abdomen
  - General effleurage
  - Ascending colon (hands in and out at 45)
  - Transverse colon (kept fingers up)
  - Descending colon (one hand lifts off and rolls off)
  - Small intestine (circles around the navel)
  - Dantain point (dan tien)
  - Right side lifts
  - Left side lifts
  - General effleurage to finish
  - Change towels

Shoulders
- Change towel
- Effleurage 3x
- Swirls in the soft spot of Décolletage
- Swirl under shoulders
- Massage neck in free flow downward moves
- Change towel

Arms
- Upper arm reverse effleurage 3x
- Inner forearm fan effleurage 3x
- Carpal stretching 3x
- Finger twist and pull with the thumb on top 3x
- Turn hand over (rotates) 3x
- Two fingers spread – soft palm kneading 3x
- Finger twist and pull. Use your fingers 3x
- Turn hand and carpal stretch3x
- Upper arm reverse effleurage 3x

Head
Can do Spa Facial, Table Shiatsu or
- ELD Face 3x each move
  - Forehead draining technique
  - Finger pressure of forehead – Rainbows
  - Forehead Drain
  - Finger pressure of forehead – Rainbows
  - Forehead Drain
  - Cheek Pressure - Rainbows
  - Cheek Drain
  - Cheek Pressure – Rainbows
  - Cheek Drain
  - Energy beside eyes
  - Chin drain
  - Forehead Drain

Finish with a foot massage.

Scalp Massage

Procedure: 5 - 30 minutes

Scalp Massage Starting Position - If the client is lying down (make sure they have a pillow under their knees).

Neck
- Support the head, turn it to one side, and hold for 30 seconds. Lightly and very slowly effleurage the neck downwards.
- Turn their head back to the center, effleurage downwards with the other hand, using the web between your finger and thumb.
- Horizontal friction along occipital ridge 3x
- Then turn to the other side and hold for 30 seconds. Lightly and very slowly effleurage the neck downwards.
- Then turn the head slowly back to the center.
- Lift forward, chin towards the chest, and hold the stretch for 30 seconds.
- Repeat 3x, using different pressure and fingers/hand.

Head
- Place the head onto the table, face up.
- Use circular motions with fingertips lightly to massage the forehead, temples, and scalp. 3-6x
- Using the fingertips, ruffle the hair all over the head 3-6x
- One hand at a time, rake the scalp 3-6x

- Lightly tapping the scalp with the fingertips—like playing a piano 3-6x
- Using both palms, lightly squeeze the scalp 3x

Swedish Massage Relaxation Routine

AN IDEA ONLY!

Once you know the basic movements, you can use the appropriate movement. Following is an example of a session.

- The client starts in the Prone position (Facedown)
- Use pillows/bolsters where necessary.
- The client's arms relaxed at their side.
- Place your hands in the resting position. Ensure your client is comfortable, gentle full body rocking over sheets.
- Palpate (sense) the client's body condition as you rock down the body.

UPPER BACK (POSTERIOR SIDE OF BODY)

Undrape the client's back *(tuck the sheet into the client's underwear if appropriate)*

1. Apply the oil by light Effleurage 2x
2. General Effleurage 3x -Checking for hot spots and the 4 T's (Tissue, Temperature, Tension/Tone, and Touch)
3. Feather stroke up back and over shoulder 3x
4. Palmer kneads - up the side of the back and shoulder 3x

5. Circles on the back, one hand or two 3x
6. Open C's over shoulder 3x
7. Thumb or use Fingertips – kneading around scapula 3x
8. Pull up over the shoulder with alternating strokes, using fingers and/or forearm 3x
9. Pull up along ribs and abdomen (caution! - avoid breast tissue) 3x
10. Walk to the other side of the table (keep contact)
11. Repeat steps on the other side of the back (A to I)
12. Play, do moves that come naturally over the entire back 3x
13. Effleurage entire back (drain lymph) 3x

LOWER BACK

14. Walk up facing head, glide both hands down towards buttocks (lightly stretch sacrum) 3x
15. Vibration down the spine and over the back 3x
16. Using the reinforced heel of the hand, do circular kneading on low back and top of the hips 3x
17. Drape the back and rub over the sheets.

BUTTOCK
Over sheet (one side at a time)

18. Ironing – sacrum (sides of hands back and forth) 3x
19. The reinforced heel of the hand 3x
20. Kneading over buttock 3x
21. Beating/pounding 3x

BACK UPPER LEGS (HAMSTRINGS)
Undrape one leg

22. Apply oil with Effleurage Stroke 3x

23. Effleurage 3x
24. Feathering up the center of the leg 3x
25. Open C's 3x
26. Kneading, Hacking, and Cupping 3x
27. Squeezing, Picking up Medial and Lateral thigh 3x
28. Shaking
29. Reinforced palmer glides up lateral side from knee to hip 3x
30. Open C's 3x
31. Effleurage 3x

BACK LOWER LEG (CALVES)

32. Effleurage 3x
33. Play
34. Alternate thumb stroking 3x
35. Wringing 3x
36. Massage foot
37. End with Effleurage of the entire leg towards the hip 3x
38. Drape the leg, and repeat this on the other leg

HAVE CLIENT TURNOVER -
Ensure the sheet fully covers the client, remove any pillows and have the client turn over onto their back (Supine).

FRONT UPPER LEGS (QUADRICEPS)
Undrape one leg

39. Apply oil with Effleurage Stroke 3x
40. Effleurage 3x
41. Open C's 3x
42. Squeezing, Picking up Medial and Lateral thigh 3x
43. Reinforced palmer glides up lateral side from knee to hip 3x
44. Effleurage 3x

FRONT LOWER LEG (SHINES)

39. Effleurage 3x
40. Alternate thumb stroking 3x
      ii)   If a calf is tight, bend the knee up and massage 3x
41. Slap their foot lightly 3x
42. Massage foot
43. End with Effleurage of the entire leg towards the hip 3x
44. Drape the leg, and repeat this on the other leg

ANTERIOR TRUNK - ABDOMEN (STOMACH)

45. Towel over the breasts and pull the sheet down towards the hips; adjust/fold the towel and sheet to reveal the stomach.
46. Oil on
47. General Effleurage (warms up the stomach to get ready for the rest of the moves)
48. The following three movements of the stomach are moving the digestive system, which runs from the person's right side to the hip at their leg, across from right to left, and then down the hip to the left side of the other leg (upside-down u-shape).
    a) The large intestine (large colon) is like an upside-down U-shape.
    b) If you go slow enough, you can sometimes feel blocked food, and it can move. This is an excellent part of the massage for healing purposes.
49. The next step is circles using both hands. (still working on the large intestine)
50. Dantain is an Energy move (waiting for the client to take a breath)
51. Side pulls and fan (is now working on getting the lymph from the back of the body to the center of the stomach)
52. General Effleurage (just relaxing the stomach after working it)

Cover up the client (you can leave a towel and pull the sheet over the top).

UPPER EXTREMITIES

Undrape one arm

53. Apply oil with Effleurage Stroke 3x
54. Effleurage 3x
55. Hold arm and palmer knead posterior side 3x
56. Feathering using thumbs up anterior of forearm 3x
57. Open C's around the shoulders 3x
58. Do hand and wrist
    massage
59. Effleurage 3x

Drape the arm, and repeat on the other arm

SHOULDER AND NECK

Reveal shoulders

60. Apply oil with Effleurage Stroke (carefully do not drip oil on face) 3x
61. Effleurage both sides same time 3x
62. Hold the head with one hand, turn to the side, glide down the lateral side of the neck, around the shoulder, and back up to the ear 3x
63. Repeat on the other side of the neck 3x
64. Turn head back to center and do Open C's down neck 3x
65. Finger circles down neck 3x
66. Effleurage 3x

HEAD AND FACE

Any ELD moves or Spa Facial if you have learned them.

67. Finger kneading from the midline of the forehead down lateral cheeks, around jawline 3x
68. Fingertip kneading over cheekbones, around lips 3x
69. Squeeze eyebrows 3x
70. Head massage, Fingertip kneading through the scalp, and effleurage off hair 3x

Table Shiatsu

TABLE SHIATSU DO'S and DON'T'S

- Apply finger pressure in a slow, rhythmic manner to enable the layers of tissues and the internal organs to respond. Never press any area in an abrupt, forceful, or jarring way.
- Use the abdominal points cautiously, especially if ill. Avoid the abdominal area entirely if the client has a life-threatening condition. Examples include intestinal cancer, TB, severe cardiac diseases, and leukemia. Also, avoid the abdominal area during pregnancy.
- Use special care during pregnancy.
- Lymph areas, such as the groin, throat below the ears, and outer breast near the armpits, are very sensitive. Touch these areas lightly and do not press.
- Do not work directly on severe burns, an ulcerative condition, varicose veins, or an infection. Medical care is indicated for these conditions.
- Do not work directly on recently formed scars. Do not apply pressure directly on the affected site during the first month after an injury or operation. Gentle continuous holding a few inches away from the periphery of the injury stimulates and encourages healing.

- After a session, the person's body heat is lowered and will have a lower resistance to the cold in the room. Vital energies are concentrated inward to maximize healing. Advise clients to dress warmly.
- Ask the client about their body and physical history. Diagnosis of a subject, from either an Oriental or Western viewpoint, is a highly complicated procedure. DO NOT DIAGNOSE. Give recommendations and suggestions. The primary purpose of Shiatsu is not to cure a disease but to help your client recover from the fatigue and strain of daily routines, relieve symptoms of a disease, or prevent it.
- Encourage your client to eat lightly before their session.
- Allow your client time to settle before commencing the session.
- Do not treat clients with broken or fractured bones. Use other modalities.
- Don't treat clients with contagious diseases; for example, flu with fever, measles, active cough, any disorders of the heart, liver, kidneys, or lungs, cancer, sarcoma, or infectious skin diseases. Serious illness has been cured by performing Shiatsu, but only by an experienced Shiatsu Therapist, with an excellent knowledge of diagnostic procedures and other forms of Oriental Medicine.
- To receive the maximum benefits, encourage the client to relax for an hour after the treatment completely. This will help to stabilize the body and encourage the flow of chi.

MERIDIANS

FIGURE 1: Anterior View of Meridians   FIGURE 2: Posterior View of Meridians

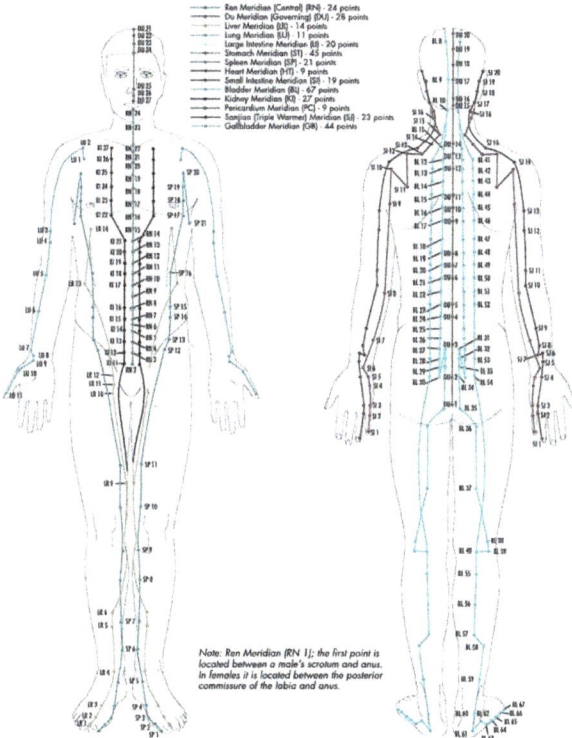

Note: Ren Meridian (RN 1); the first point is located between a male's scrotum and anus. In females it is located between the posterior commissure of the labia and anus.

CONSTANCE SANTEGO.CA
Shift happens... Create magic!

SHIATSU PROCEDURE

BACK (Prone)

(Standing on the client's left side)

- Stand beside the client and bring Chi to your hands. Center yourself, focus your intent, touch the client, and begin to sense the receiver.
- Palm shiatsu down the left side of the spine.
- Palm shiatsu down the right side of the spine.
- Cross arms. Place one hand on the iliac crest (lower back) and the other on the opposite scapula. Lean using light body weight. Switch hands (sides) and repeat.
- Cup the spine and gently rock the spine from side to side moving down to the sacrum. Repeat.

(Standing at the head of the table)

- Run hands down the inner Bladder- BL meridian to the waist and bilaterally brush hands up the body, neck, and over the crown of the head. Repeat.
- Thumb shiatsu up the inner BL meridian from the waist to the top of the shoulders.
- Glide hands up the neck to GB20 (follow the neck up to the scull, 1" above).
- Hold GB20 (follow the neck up to scull, 1" above) with fingertips and lean backward. This applies light traction to the neck. Repeat.
- Hold BL10 (C1) with fingertips and then inchworm up the scalp pressing points along the BL meridian.
- Squeeze scalp.

- Hold GB21 (soft spot on shoulders) with your thumbs while finger pressing SI points on the scapular plate (top of scapula SI 12, lateral side of SI 10, and the middle point of SI 11 (Triangle). Repeat.
- Squeeze trapezius.
- Run hands down the inner BL meridian to the waist and bilaterally brush hands up the body, neck, and over the crown of the head. Repeat.
- Thumb shiatsu up the inner BL meridian from the waist to the top of the shoulders. (20 points)
- Glide hands up the neck to GB20 (on the head).
- Hold GB20 (on the head) with your fingertips and lean backward. This applies light traction to the neck. Repeat.
- Hold BL10 (C1) with fingertips and then inchworm up the scalp pressing points along the BL meridian.
- Squeeze scalp.

(Standing on the client's left side)

- Hold Lu1 (the soft spot where the arm and shoulder meet) with your yin hand.
- Forearm roll along the upper trapezius. x 3
- Forearm roll out the scapula. x 3
- Elbow shiatsu SI 9 (on the back, a soft spot above the scapula, on the arm/shoulder). x 3
- Thumb shiatsu SI (top of scapula SI 12, lateral side SI 10- and middle-point SI 11 (Triangle) points on the scapular plate.
- Forearm roll along the upper trapezius. x 3
- Forearm roll out the scapula. x 3
- Forearm press the ribs.
- Elbow shiatsu the sacrum points. BL 36 BL 33, BL 53
- Forearm roll down the back. Repeat x 2.
- Elbow shiatsu the sacrum points. BL 36 BL 33, BL 53

- Forearm roll down the back. Repeat x 2.

(Standing on the client's right side)

- Repeat shoulder and torso work on the client's right side.

(Standing on the client's right side)

- Palm lean on BL 54 (both sides)
- Squeeze sacrum.
- Repeat.

(Position yourself at the foot of the table)

Both Left and Right feet at the same time

- Hold K 3 (inside ankle) and BL 60 (outside ankle) and lean back to apply light traction. Release traction and gently shake legs to release hips.
- Press legs inward at ankles.
- Press legs outward and down at ankles.
- Press fists into arches of feet.
- Thumb shiatsu down yang side of feet.
- Thumb shiatsu down the middle of feet.
- Thumb shiatsu down yin side of feet.
- Hold K 3 and BL 60 (either side of the ankle) and lean back to apply light traction.

LEFT LEG

- Squeeze the calf from K 3 and BL 60 (either side of the ankle) to the knee.
- Slide your hand down the calf to KI 3 and BL60 (either side of the ankle) and give the leg a slight pull.
- Hold the knee crease with your yin hand and rotate the leg in slow circles. Reverse.
- Place the left forearm increase of the knee and fold the foot towards the buttocks.
- Move the forearm to mid-thigh and repeat.
- Move the forearm to the top of the thigh and repeat.
- Place the leg in a bent position (the knee towards you, flat on the table) and palm press from the hip to the ankle, down the GB meridian on the side of the leg (GB30 to GB41).
- ****Straighten the leg and place your hands on either side of the knee.
- Palm pressure with both hands along the BL meridian until one hand is at the gluteus ridge (BL54) and the other is at the ankle (BL60). Then, stretch the leg with both hands. **NEVER apply pressure directly on the knee.**

RIGHT LEG

- Repeat on the left leg.

(Position yourself at the foot of the client)

- Hold the K 3 and BL 60 (either side of the ankle) and lean back to apply light traction. Release traction and gently shake the legs to release the hips.
- Apply firm thumb shiatsu in K 1 (sole of foot, reflex point solar plexus).
- Energy sweeps down the legs.

FRONT (Supine) Turn the client over, face-up

(Position yourself at the right foot of the client)

- Hold K 3 and BL 60 meridian (either side of the ankle).
- Ankle range of motion (circles).
- Lean (towards the client) and pull the foot (away from the client) x 3.
- Thumb shiatsu up the yin side of the foot.
- Thumb shiatsu up the middle of the foot.
- Pinch up yang the side of the foot.
- Glide your thumb up the yin side of the foot.
- Glide thumbs/fingers in a circular motion around the ankles.
- Lightly rotate and pull each toe.
- Ankle range of motion (circles).
- Lean and pull the foot x 3.
- Fan the toes.

(Stand on the client's right leg)

- Leg range (SP, LR and KI). Expose the inside of the leg by bending it at (the ankle, mid-calf, and knee), and palm press from hip to ankle in each position.
- Pick up the leg and bend it at the knee. Then, rotate the leg at the hip socket <u>outwards</u> (3 circles, small to large).
- Press the leg towards the chest.
- Rotate the leg at the hip socket <u>inwards</u> (3 circles, small to large).
- Press the leg towards the chest.
- Hold GB30 (hip) and gently shakedown the GB meridian to GB41 (midfoot).

(Position yourself at the left foot of the client)

Repeat the front foot and leg routine on the left leg.

(Position yourself at the end of the table)

- Hold above ankles and lean back to apply light traction. Release traction lifts slightly and gently shakes legs to release hips (Fallen Leaf).
- Energy sweeps down legs.

ABDOMEN

(Position yourself on the client's right side)

- Stroking (soothing, brushing)
- Diamond glide under ribs with a side of the hand, slide fingers behind back, then up to gently pinch navel. Repeat.
- Stroke the abdomen in a circular, hand-over-hand clockwise motion. x 9
- Support back (under them) with Yin hand and thumb shiatsu down Conception Vessel (center / Ren). Coordinate shiatsu with abdominal breathing.
- With both hands, thumb shiatsu down ST meridian. Coordinate shiatsu with abdominal breathing.
- Diamond glide under ribs with a side of the hand, slide fingers behind back, then up to gently pinch navel. Repeat.
- Vibrate the navel and lift quickly to seal the chi.

ARMS

(Client's right arm)

- Palm leans into LU 1 (the front soft spot where the arm and shoulder meet)
- Squeeze down the arm from the shoulder to the fingertips.

(Expose Yin side of the client's right arm)

Hold source points LU 9, PC 7, HT 7 (inside wrists)

- Palm or thumb shiatsu down the LU meridian. (Thumb)
- Palm or thumb shiatsu down the PC meridian. (Middle)
- Palm or thumb shiatsu down the HT meridian. (Pinky)

(Expose Yang side of the client's right arm)

Hold source points SI 4, SJ/TW 4, LI 4 (back of wrists)

- Palm or thumb shiatsu down the SI meridian. (Pinky)
- Palm or thumb shiatsu down the SJ/TW meridian. (Ring finger)
- Palm or thumb shiatsu down the LI meridian. (Pointer)

HANDS

(Open the client's right hand by hooking your little fingers behind the client's thumb and little finger)

- Stroke the palm with your thumbs.
- Thumb shiatsu up the palm in three lines.
- Stroke the palm with your thumbs.
- Expose the Yang side of the hand.

- Release the wrist points. (hold each side of the wrist and shake back and forth)
- Rotate and pull each finger.
- Put your fingers between the clients, rotate their wrists, and lightly stretch the joint.
- Hold the wrist with one hand and elbow with the other, then rotate the elbow in both directions.
- Shake and stretch the arm in 4 positions.
  - By their side,
  - out towards you,
  - up towards the ceiling
  - then past their head.
- Return the arm to the client's side.
- Hold GB 21 (shoulder) and lightly pull the arm towards their feet.

(Stand on the client's left side)

- Repeat ARMS and HANDS on the client's left side.

SHOULDERS

(Position yourself at the crown of the client)

- Depress the shoulders at LU 1 by using your body weight (fingers facing out)
- Depress the shoulders at LU 1 by using your body weight (fingers facing in)
- Depress the shoulders at LU 1 by using your body weight (fingers facing down)
- While holding the client's head with your yin hand (under the head).
  - Apply thumb pressure to GB21 (shoulder ridge).

- o Apply thumb and finger pressure on the head – BL10 to BL2. (the points you did when you inchworm)
  - o Apply pressure to GB14 (mid-forehead above the eyes).
- Stretch the right side of their neck (place your arm under their neck (their head is resting on the posterior side of your arm). Using one arm, your fingertips should be on the anterior side of one of their shoulders, while your elbow should be near the other shoulder. Press the points on the base of the skull (BL10 (C1 (inside), and GB20 (outside and up)
- Repeat on the left side of the neck.

FACE

- Sooth the points across the forehead.
- Lightly squeeze the upper eyebrow.
- Very lightly apply pressure under the eye sockets.
- Apply pressure with fingertips under cheekbones. Focus on ST 3(check bone, either side of the nose) "Facial Beauty."
- Thumb shiatsu above the mouth and out to the ears. Roll the ears back and lightly pull.
- Thumb shiatsu below the mouth.
- Apply pressure with your fingertips under the chin.
- Hold GB20 (scull) with your fingertips and lean backward. This applies light traction to the neck. Gently return their head to the table.
- Lightly touch
  - o DU/GV20 "One Hundred Meeting Point" (Crown chakra) with your yin hand while touching points below with your yang hand. One at a time.
  - o RN/CV17 (Heart chakra) "Sea of Tranquility"
  - o RN/CV22 (Throat charka) "Heaven Rushing Out"

o   DU/GV24.5 (Brow charka) "Third Eye Point"
     with yang hand.

This connects their heart, body, and mind.

End the session

- Stroke the "Never Ending Hand" down their forehead and over their crown. Repeat.
- Place both palms gently over their eyes and end the session. Then, in your mind, give thanks.
- Allow the client a peaceful, sacred moment.

TIPS and TRICKS
to having a pain free body

1st secret...

> **Goldi Tendon Organ Release Technique**
> (push and hold for the count of ten)
>
> Shoulder: rub around the shoulder blade, end of the shoulder, and collar bone (u-shape motion)
>
> Arm: also rub around the shoulder blade, end of the shoulder, and collar bone (u-shape motion)
>
> Butt: rub the edge of the hip to tail bone or apply pressure with all fingers
>
> Leg: Calf muscle tightness or cramps *at Achilles heel (calcaneal tendon) and just below the knee, soleus origin attachment*
>
> > Anterior calf muscles (tibialis anterior-medial and peroneals -lateral)
> >
> > *= at the base of the first metatarsal*
> >
> > Hamstrings (back of the leg) *ischial tuberosity (sit bone)*
> >
> > Quadriceps (front of the leg) *rectus femoris, just above the knee and at the crease of the leg*
> >
> > *= all other anterior thigh muscles, just above the knee*

Foot:

> Flexor Digitorum Brevis (Plantar fasciitis) *at the edge of the calcaneus bone or the pad of the toes*

2nd secret...

Agonist Contract - Opposite Muscle Technique (*remedial exercise-AIH*)

Move your body in the opposite direction of the movement that causes the pain. Don't forget to apply light pressure and count to five.

3rd secret...

Epsom salts

> Magnesium is excellent for relaxing muscles, and the other part of the salt helps to flush lactic acid and waste caused by muscle use (1 cup in warm to hot water for 20 minutes min).

4th secret...

Stretch in shower

> After you have cleansed yourself, let the warm hot water massage your neck and let your neck flex at its speed (do not force it), then let the water hit your back and allow each vertebra to relax, watch how fast you can touch your toes without effort.

5th secret...

Quick Fix

Rubbing all the neuro-lymphatic points three times. Go to my website for a copy of the diagram and instructions on how to do it. www.constancesantego.ca

6th secret...

Meditation

Go to my YouTube Channel - *Constance Santego,* and listen to the different meditations. Find one that works for you. Then, spend at least two times a week meditating, daily if possible.

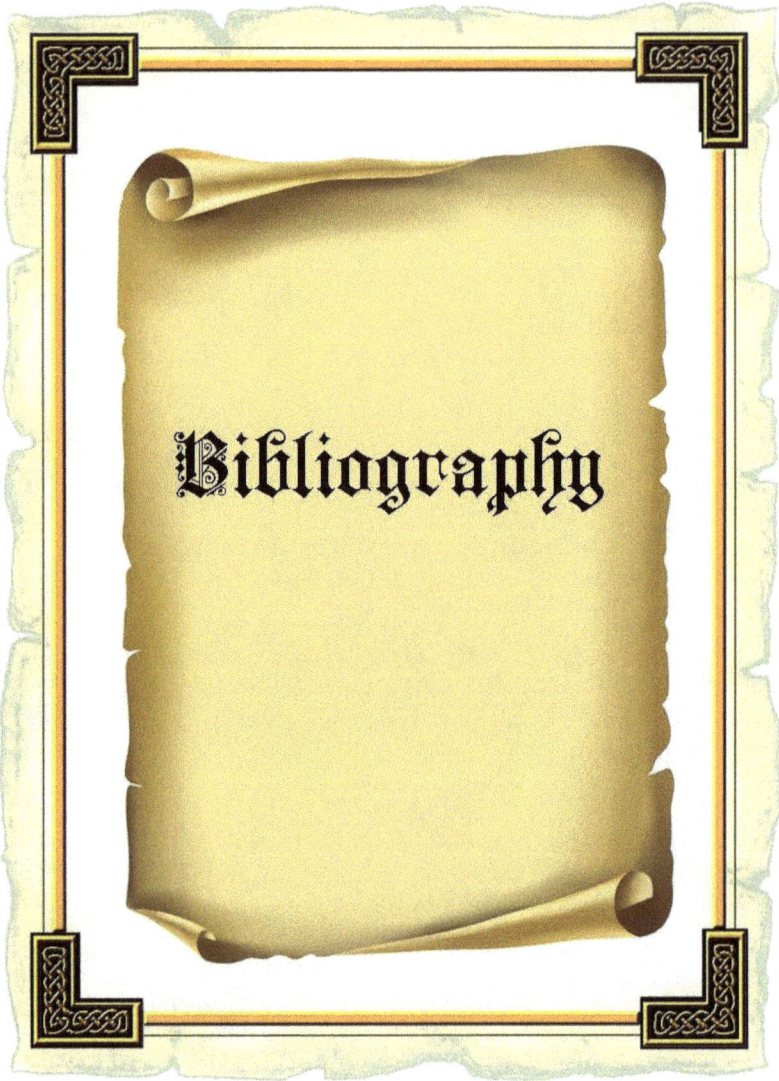

Bibliography

Much of this information was taken from the course information created when I owned the Canadian Institute of Natural Health and Healing Accredited College.

Lyle J. Micheli, M.D. (1995) The Sports Medicine Bible. Harper Perennial

Mel Cash (1996) Sport and Remedial Massage Therapy. Edbury Press

Gregory Pike (1997) Sports Massage for Peak Performance. Harper Perennial

Mark F. Beck (2002) Massage Basics, A guide to Swedish, Shiatsu, and Reflexology Techniques. Delmar

Jacqueline Young (1992) Self-Massage, The complete 15-minute-a-day Massage Programme

Peijian Shen (1996) Massage for pain relief, a step-by-step guide

Joesph and Sandra Duggan (1995) Edgar Cayce's Massage Hydrotherapy and Healing Oils

Stewart Mitchell (1997) Massage, A Practical Introduction

Nigel Dawes and Fiona Harrold (1990) Massage Cures, the family guide to curing common ailments with simple massage techniques

Muriel Burnham-Airey and Adele O'Keefe (2005) Indian head massage

MASSAGE THERAPY TEXTBOOKS:

Susan G. Salvo (2014) Mosby's Pathology, for Massage Therapists, third edition

Luigi Stecco (2004) Facial Manipulation for Musculoskeletal pain
Abby Ellsworth Dr. and Peggy Altman (2009) Massage Anatomy

Donna Fiando (2005) Trigger Point Therapy for Myofascial Pain

Chris Jarmey (2008) The Concise Book of Muscles, second edition

Alfred F. Morris (1985) Sports Medicine Handbook

Clair Davies (2004) The Trigger Point Therapy Workbook, second edition

Andrew Biel (2014) Trail Guide to the Body

Bob Anderson (2010) Stretching

David j. Magee (2014) Orthopedic Physical Assessment, sixth edition

Susan G. Salvo (1999) Massage Therapy principles and practice

Fiona Rattray (2000) Clinical Massage Therapy

Castor Oil

https://www.healthline.com/nutrition/castor-oil

https://www.tipsbulletin.com/castor-oil-uses-and-benefits/

https://www.goodhousekeeping.com/beauty/a20707265/castor-oil-uses/

Message From The Author

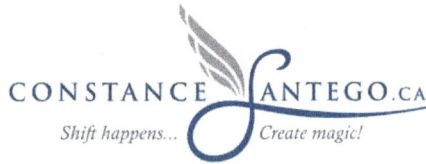

It has been over twenty years, and I still love massage. Touch is one of the most intimate and bonding rituals a person can do.

Now that I have retired from teaching these courses. I decided I didn't want the knowledge to go to waste, and here you have it. I have gifted you the massages that I taught to my Holistic, Natural Health, Day Spa, and Esthetician students.

Play and have fun learning these marvelously relaxing and beneficial massages.

From my heart to yours, enjoy!

Constance

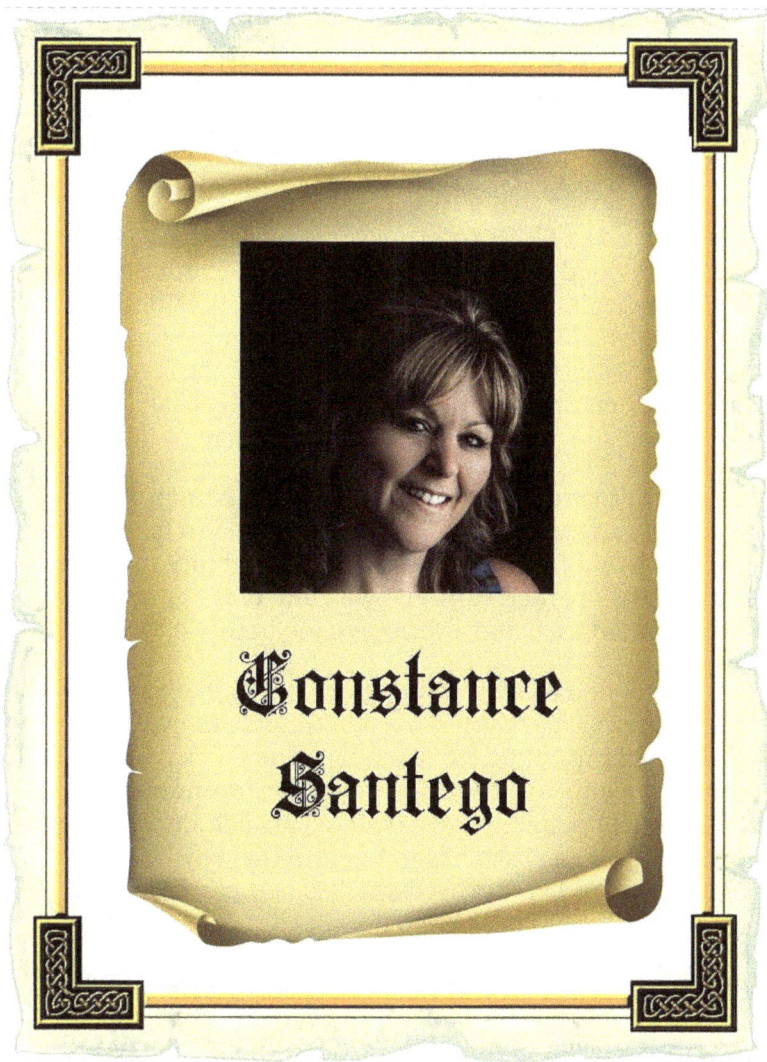

Constance Santego

Shift happens...Create magic!
Dream BIGGER!

Dr. Constance Santego is a highly respected expert in the field of holistic health and spiritual healing. With over twenty years of experience teaching courses on these subjects, she has developed a deep understanding of the interconnectedness of the mind, body, and spirit in achieving overall well-being.

Dr. Santego holds a Ph.D. and Doctorate in Natural Medicine, which has provided her with a comprehensive understanding of alternative healing modalities and their application in promoting optimal health. Her educational background has equipped her with the knowledge to address health concerns from a holistic perspective, considering the physical, emotional, and spiritual aspects of an individual's well-being.

Throughout her career, Dr. Santego has been committed to sharing her knowledge and empowering others to take control of their health and healing. She has a unique ability to blend scientific research and traditional wisdom, creating a bridge between conventional and alternative medicine.

In her "Secrets of a Healer" educational series, Dr. Santego draws upon her vast experience and expertise to captivate readers with her insights and teachings. She takes readers on a transformative journey, delving into the realms of holistic health, spirituality, and self-discovery. Through her writing, she aims to inspire individuals to tap into their own innate healing abilities and embrace a balanced and harmonious approach to well-being.

Dr. Santego's work has touched the lives of many, guiding them toward a more profound understanding of themselves and their connection to the world around them. Her series serves as a beacon of wisdom, offering practical tools and techniques for personal growth and transformation.

Overall, Dr. Constance Santego's blend of knowledge, experience, and passion makes her a captivating figure in the field of holistic health and spiritual healing. Her contributions through teaching, writing, and her spellbinding series continue to inspire and empower individuals on their journeys toward well-being and self-discovery.

ALSO AVAILABLE

Play the game *Ikona* – Discover Your Inner Genie

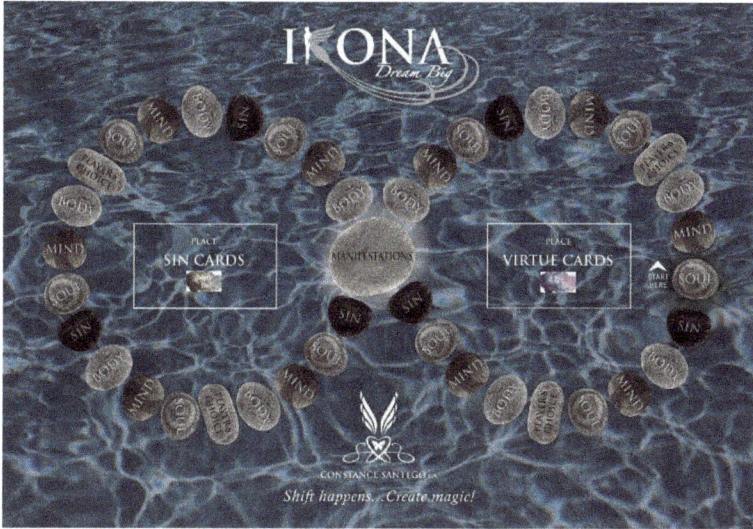

For additional information on

Constance Santego's

wide range of Motivational Products, Coaching Sessions,
Spiritual Retreats,
Live Events and Educational Programs

Go to

www.ConstanceSantego.ca

Follow on Instagram - Constance_Santego and
Facebook - constancesantegoo

Subscribe and receive Free Information and Meditations
on my
YouTube Channel - Constance Santego